Fish's Clinical Psychopathology

Signs and symptoms in psychiatry

D1338796

Third edition

Patricia Casey and Brendan Kelly

Gaskell

This edition © The Royal College of Psychiatrists 2007.
Reprinted 2008, with amendments.
Reprinted 2009, 2011.
Previous editions © John Wright & Sons Ltd.

Gaskell is an imprint of the Royal College of Psychiatrists,
17 Belgrave Square, London SW1X 8PG
http://www.rcpsych.ac.uk

British Library Cataloguing-in-Publication Data.
A catalogue record for this book is available from the British Library.
ISBN-10   1 904671 32 2
ISBN-13   978 1 904671 32 9

Distributed in North America by Publishers Storage and Shipping Comany.

The views presented in this book do not necessarily reflect those of the Royal College of Psychiatrists, and the publishers are not responsible for any error of omission or fact.

The Royal College of Psychiatrists is a charity registered in England and Wales (228636) and in Scotland (SC038369).

Printed by Bell & Bain Limited, Glasgow, UK.

Contents

The authors

Patricia Casey is Professor of Psychiatry at University College Dublin and Consultant Psychiatrist at Mater Misericordiae University Hospital, School of Medicine and Medical Science, Eccles Street, Dublin 7, Ireland

Brendan Kelly is Consultant Psychiatrist and Senior Lecturer in Psychiatry, Department of Adult Psychiatry, University College Dublin, Mater Misericordiae University Hospital, Dublin, Ireland

Preface

Psychopathology is the science and study of psychological and psychiatric symptoms. Clinical psychopathology locates this study in the clinical context in which psychiatrists make diagnostic assessments and deliver mental health services. A clear understanding of clinical psychopathology lies at the heart of effective and appropriate delivery of such services.

In 1967, Frank Fish produced a 128-page volume on psychopathology, entitled *Clinical Psychopathology: Signs and Symptoms in Psychiatry* (Fish, 1967). Despite its brevity or more likely, because of its brevity, *Fish's Clinical Psychopathology* soon became an essential text for medical students, psychiatric trainees and all healthcare workers involved in the delivery of mental health services. A revised edition, edited by Max Hamilton, appeared in 1974 (Hamilton, 1974) and was reprinted as a second edition in 1985 (Hamilton, 1985).

In recent years, *Fish's Clinical Psychopathology* has been out of print and essentially impossible to locate. The purpose of this third edition is to introduce this classic text to a new generation of psychiatrists and trainees, and to reacquaint existing aficionados with the elegant insights and enduring values of Fish's original work.

Revising *Fish's Clinical Psychopathology* has been both a humbling and exciting experience. While striving at all times to retain the spirit of Fish's original work, we have revised the language in various areas so as to take account of changes in linguistic conventions. We have also updated references and included new material relating to personality disorder, cognitive distortion, defence mechanisms, memory and unusual psychiatric syndromes.

Notwithstanding these revisions, we trust that this text remains true to the spirit of Fish's original *Clinical Psychopathology*, the volume that shaped the clinical education and practice of a generation of psychiatrists. We hope that this edition proves similarly useful to contemporary readers. If it succeeds, all credit lies with the original insights of Frank Fish; if it does not, the fault lies with us.

Patricia Casey
Brendan Kelly

References

Fish, F. (1967) *Clinical Psychopatholgy: Signs and Symptoms in Psychiatry*. Bristol: John Wright & Sons.

Hamilton, M. (ed.) (1974) *Fish's Clinical Psychopathology: Signs and Symptoms in Psychiatry* (revised edn). Bristol: John Wright & Sons.

Hamilton, M. (ed.) (1985) *Fish's Clinical Psychopathology: Signs and Symptoms in Psychiatry* (2nd edn). Bristol: John Wright & Sons.

CHAPTER 1

Classification of psychiatric disorders

Any discussion of the classification of psychiatric disorders should begin with the frank admission that the definitive classification of disease must be based on aetiology. Until we know the cause of the various mental illnesses, we must adopt a pragmatic approach to classification that will best enable us to care for our patients, to communicate with other health professionals and to carry out high-quality research.

In physical medicine, syndromes existed long before the aetiology of these illnesses were known. Some of these syndromes have subsequently been shown to be true disease entities because they have one essential cause. Thus, smallpox and measles were carefully described and differentiated by the Arabian physician Rhazes in the 10th century AD. With each new step in the progress of medicine, such as auscultation, microscopy, immunology, electrophysiology, etc., some syndromes have been found to be true disease entities, while others have been split into more discrete entities and others jettisoned. For example, diabetes mellitus has been shown to be a syndrome that can have several different aetiologies. On that basis the modern approach to classification has been to establish syndromes in order to facilitate research and to assist us in extending our knowledge of them so that ultimately specific diseases can be identified. We must not forget that syndromes may or may not be true disease entities and some will argue that the multifactorial aetiology of psychiatric disorder, related to both constitutional and environmental vulnerability, as well as to precipitants, may make the goal of identifying psychiatric syndromes as discrete diseases an elusive ideal.

Syndromes and diseases

A syndrome is a constellation of symptoms that are unique as a group. It may of course contain some symptoms that occur in other syndromes also, but it is the particular combination of symptoms that makes the syndrome specific. In psychiatry, as in other branches of medicine, many syndromes began as one specific and striking symptom. In the 19th century, stupor, furore and hallucinosis were syndromes based on one prominent symptom.

Later, the recognition that certain other signs and symptoms co-occurred simultaneously led to the establishment of true syndromes. Korsakoff's syndrome illustrates the progression from symptom to syndrome to disease. Initially, confabulation and impressibility among alcoholics were recognised by Korsakoff as significant symptoms. Later the presence of disorientation for time and place, euphoria, difficulty in registration, confabulation and 'tram-line' thinking were identified as key features of this syndrome. Finally, the discovery that in the alcoholic amnestic syndrome there was always severe damage to the mammillary bodies confirmed that Korsakoff's psychosis (syndrome) is a true disease with a neuropathological basis.

Sometimes the symptoms of the syndrome seem to have a meaningful coherence. For example, in mania the cheerfulness, the overactivity, the pressure of speech and the flight of ideas can all be understood as arising from the elevated mood. The fact that we can empathise with and understand our patients' symptoms has led to the distinction between those symptoms that are primary and which are said to be the immediate result of the disease process, and secondary symptoms, which are a psychological elaboration of, or reaction to, primary symptoms. The term is also used to describe symptoms that cannot be derived from any other psychological event.

Early distinctions

The first major classification of mental illness was based on the distinction between disorders arising from disease of the brain and those with no such obvious basis, i.e. organic versus functional states. These terms are still used, but as knowledge of the neurobiological processes associated with psychiatric disorders has increased, their original meaning has been lost. Schizophrenia and manic depression are typical examples of functional disorders, but the increasing evidence of the role of genetics and of neuropathological abnormalities shows that there is at least some organic basis for these disorders. Indeed the category of 'organic mental syndromes and disorders' has been renamed as 'delirium, dementia and amnestic and other cognitive disorders' in the *Diagnostic and Statistical Manual of Mental Disorders* (DSM)–IV (American Psychiatric Association, 1994), so that the recognition of the role of abnormal brain functioning is not confined to dementia and delirium only. In their literal meaning these categories of classification (i.e. organic versus functional) are absurd, yet they continue to be used through tradition.

Organic syndromes

The syndromes due to brain disorders can be classified into acute, subacute and chronic. In acute organic syndromes the most common feature is alteration of consciousness, which can be dream-like, depressed or restricted. This gives rise to four subtypes, i.e. delirium, subacute delirium, organic stupor or torpor, and the twilight state. Disorientation, incoherence of psychic life and some degree of anterograde amnesia are features of all of these acute organic states. In delirium there is a dream-like change in consciousness so that the patient may also be unable to distinguish between mental images and perceptions, leading to hallucinations and illusions. Usually there is severe anxiety and agitation. When stupor or torpor is established the patient responds poorly or not at all to stimuli and after recovery has no recollection of events during the episode. In subacute delirium there is a general lowering of awareness and marked incoherence of psychic activity, so that the patient is bewildered and perplexed. Isolated hallucinations, illusions and delusions may occur and the level of awareness varies but is lower at night-time. The subacute delirious state can be regarded as a transitional state between delirium and organic stupor. In twilight states consciousness is restricted, so that the mind is dominated by a small group of ideas, attitudes and images. These patients may appear to be perplexed but often their behaviour is well ordered and they can carry out complex actions. Hallucinations are commonly present. In organic stupor (torpor) the level of consciousness is generally lowered and the patient responds poorly or not at all to stimuli. After recovery the patient usually has amnesia for the events that occurred during the illness episode.

In addition to the above, there are organic syndromes in which consciousness is not obviously disordered, for example organic hallucinosis due to alcohol abuse, which is characterised by hallucinations, most commonly auditory and occurring in clear consciousness, as distinct from the hallucinations of delirium tremens that occur in association with clouded consciousness. Amnestic disorders, of which Korsakoff's syndrome is but one, also belong in this group of organic disorders and are characterised primarily by the single symptom of memory impairment in a setting of clear consciousness and in the absence of other cognitive features of dementia.

The chronic organic states include the various dementias, generalised and focal, as well as the amnestic disorders. Included among the generalised dementias are Lewy body disease, Alzheimer's disease, etc., while the best known focal dementia is frontal lobe dementia (or syndrome). The latter is associated with a lack of drive, lack of foresight, inability to plan ahead and an indifference to the feelings of others, although there is no disorientation. Some patients may also demonstrate a happy-go-lucky carelessness and a facetious humour, termed *Witzelsucht*, whereas others are rigid in their thinking and have difficulty moving from one topic to the next. The most common cause is trauma to the brain such as occurs in road traffic accidents. The presence of frontal lobe damage may be assessed psychologically using the Wisconsin Card Sorting test or the Stroop test. Amnestic disorders are chronic organic disorders in which there is the single symptom of memory impairment; if other signs of cognitive impairment are present (such as disorientation or impaired attention) the diagnosis is dementia. The major neuroanatomical structures involved are the thalamus, hippocampus, mammillary bodies and the amygdala. Amnesia is usually the result of bilateral damage but some cases can occur with unilateral damage and the left hemisphere appears to be more critical than the right in its genesis.

Functional syndromes

Functional disorders, a phrase seldom used nowadays, refers to those syndromes in which there is no readily-apparent coarse brain disease, although increasingly it is recognised that some finer variety of brain disease may exist, often at a cellular level.

For many years it was customary to divide these functional mental illnesses into neuroses and psychoses. The person with neurosis was believed to have insight into his illness, with only part of his personality involved in the disorder, and to have intact reality testing. The individual with psychosis, on the other hand, was believed to lack insight, had the whole of his personality distorted by the illness and constructed a false environment out of his distorted subjective experience. However, such differences are an oversimplification, since many individuals with neurotic conditions have no insight, and far from accepting their illness, may minimise or deny it totally, while people with schizophrenia may seek help willingly during or before episodes of relapse. Moreover, personality can be changed significantly by non-psychotic disorders such as depressive illness, while it may be intact in some people with psychotic disorders such as persistent delusional disorder.

Jaspers (1962) regarded the person with neurosis as an individual who has an abnormal response to difficulties in which some specific defence mechanism has transformed their experiences. For example, in conversion and dissociative disorders (formerly hysteria) the mechanism of dissociation is used to transform the emotional experiences into physical symptoms. Since we can all use this mechanism, the differences between the neurotic person and the normal person is one of degree. Schneider (1959) has suggested the neuroses and personality disorders are variations of human existence that differ from the norm quantitatively rather than qualitatively. However, this view of the neuroses breaks down when obsessive–compulsive disorder is considered, since the symptoms are not variations of normal but differ qualitatively from normal behaviours.

Over time the use of the terms neurotic and psychotic changed and instead of describing symptoms, particularly symptom types such as hallucinations or delusions, in the psychotic person they were used to distinguish mild and severe disorders or to distinguish those symptoms that were ego-syntonic (i.e. creating no distress for the person or compatible with the indiviudal's self-concept or ego) or ego-dystonic (i.e. causing distress and incompatible with the person's self-concept). Some practitioners also used the word 'neurotic' as a term of opprobrium. Owing to the confusion that abounded in the various uses of these terms, DSM−IV has excluded the term 'neurosis' totally from its nomenclature and International Classification of Diseases (ICD) − 10 (World Health Organization, 1992) has limited its use to a group of disorders entitled 'neurotic, stress-related and somatoform disorders'.

Personality disorders and psychogenic reactions

The status of personality disorder vis-à-vis other psychiatric disorders was historically regarded differently in the English-speaking world compared with the rest of the world. In the English-speaking world, it was customary to separate the neuroses from personality disorders, but in the German-speaking countries, epitomised by Schneider, the neuroses were regarded as reactions of abnormal personalities to moderate or mild stress and of normal personalities to severe stress. This difference in approach continues and is reflected in the differing approaches to personality disorder in DSM and ICD, with the former placing personality disorder on a separate axis from other disorders, while ICD–10 represents both on Axis I (see below).

Psychogenic reactions constituted reversible prolonged psychological responses to trauma, the reactions being the consequence of the causative agent on the patient's personality. Thus acute anxiety and hysteria were considered to be varieties of psychogenic reactions provoked by stress and determined by personality and cultural factors. Sometimes the stress was believed to cause psychotic reactions, termed symptomatic or psychogenic psychoses; for example the person with a paranoid personality who, in light of ongoing marital difficulties, begins to suspect his wife's fidelity, finally becoming deluded about this. The idea of delusional states that were not due to functional psychoses was treated with skepticism by English-speaking psychiatrists, but had adherents in Scandinavia, particularly in what were termed psychogenic psychoses. These have gained increasing acceptance and are now called acute and transient psychotic disorders in ICD–10 and brief psychotic disorder with or without marked stressors in DSM–IV.

In summary, Schneider (1959) considered that neuroses, psychogenic reactions and personality disorders were not illnesses in the sense that there was a morbid process in the nervous system, while he considered that functional psychoses did represent true illnesses.

Modern classifications

The 4th edition of the DSM (DSM–IV) (American Psychiatric Association, 1994) is the most recently published classification of mental disorders, although there has been a more recent text revision of the manual, entitled DSM–IV–TR (2000). DSM–IV is used in the USA and notwithstanding the fact that the World Health Organization has developed the 10th edition of the ICD (ICD–10) (World Health Organization, 1992), the latter has found little usage in the USA, although it remains the main classification used in Britain, Ireland and almost the whole of Europe.

DSM–I, published by the American Psychiatric Association, first appeared in 1952 and since then it has evolved significantly, to the extent that DSM–IV includes large amounts of detail concerning each syndrome and, owing to its rigorous adherence to operational definitions for each disorder, it is suitable for use in both clinical practice and research. For this reason

DSM−IV is considerably less user-friendly than ICD−10 and is also considered excessively procrustean by its critics. Interestingly, the billing codes for Medicare in the USA are mandated to follow the ICD system rather than their own DSM−IV.

ICD−10 on the other hand is more clinically orientated and is not so rigid in its definitions, eschewing operational definitions in favour of general descriptions. It allows clinical judgement to inform diagnoses, but this freedom makes it unsuitable for research purposes, necessitating the development of separate research diagnostic criteria. Thus, different versions of ICD−10 now exist and these include the clinical version (World Health Organization, 1992), a version with diagnostic criteria for research (World Health Organization, 1993) (which resembles DSM in its use of detailed operational criteria) and a version for use in primary care (ICD−10−PC; World Health Organization, 1996), the latter consisting of definitions for 25 common conditions as well as a shorter version of 6 disorders for use by other primary care workers. Management guidelines incorporate information for the patient as well as details of medical, social and psychological interventions. Finally, assistance on when to refer for specialist treatment is provided.

DSM−IV also has a primary care version (DSM−IV−PC) that is similar to ICD−10−PC, focusing on the most common disorders seen in primary care (anxiety, depression, substance misuse, etc.).

Although both ICD−10 and DSM−IV are broadly similar, the language used to describe each disorder differs significantly. The differences, both in general approach and in language, are illustrated in the descriptions of depressive episode (see Boxes 1.1 and 1.2).

Comparison of DSM−IV and ICD−10

It is important to recognise that DSM−IV and ICD−10 are syndrome-based classifications, but as our knowledge increases, some classifications currently included may be removed or new categories may be added. For example, depressive personality disorder is not included in ICD−10 and is only incorporated in the section of DSM−IV entitled 'Criteria sets and axes provided for further study'. On the other hand, passive−aggressive personality disorder was included in DSM−III but excluded from the subsequent edition, and has never been incorporated into the ICD system.

ICD−10 does not distinguish bipolar I and II disorder, as does DSM−IV, as these conditions have only come to be recognised in the 1990s. Recurrent brief depressive disorder is a new addition to ICD−10 but only appears in the appendix of DSM−IV. Schizotypal disorder is classified with the schizophrenic disorders in ICD−10 and with the personality disorders in DSM−IV. Any belief, therefore, that the categories incorporated in either system of classification are 'writ in stone' is deeply misplaced.

There are also differences in the number of axes used (see below) in each and in the level of operational definition (as mentioned above).

Box 1.1 DSM–IV–TR Criteria for major depressive episode (American Psychiatric Association, 2000. Reprinted by permission of the American Psychiatric Association, © 2000).

DSM–IV–TR Criteria for Major Depressive Episode

A. Five (or more) of the following symptoms have been present during the same 2-week period and represent a change from previous functioning; at least one of the symptoms is either (1) depressed mood or (2) loss of interest or pleasure.

Note: Do not include symptoms that are clearly due to a general medical condition, or mood-incongruent delusions or hallucinations.

(1) depressed mood most of the day, nearly every day, as indicated by either subjective report (e.g., feels sad or empty) or observation made by others (e.g., appears tearful). Note: in children or adolescents, can be irritable mood

(2) markedly diminished interest or pleasure in all, or almost all, activities of the day, nearly every day (as indicated by either subjective account or observation made by others)

(3) significant weight loss when not dieting or weight gain (e.g., a change of more than 5% of body weight in a month), or decrease or increase in appetite nearly every day. Note: In children, consider failure to make expected weight gains

(4) insomnia or hypersomnia nearly every day

(5) psychomotor agitation or retardation nearly every day (observable by others, not merely subjective feelings of restlessness or being slowed down)

(6) fatigue or loss of energy nearly every day

(7) feelings of worthlessness or excessive or inappropriate guilt (which may be delusional) nearly every day (not merely self-reproach or guilt about being sick)

(8) diminished ability to think or concentrate, or indecisiveness, nearly every day (either by subjective account or as observed by others)

(9) recurrent thoughts of death (not just fear of dying), recurrent suicidal ideation without a specific plan, or a suicide attempt or a specific plan for committing suicide

B. The symptoms do not meet criteria for a Mixed Episode (see p. 365)

C. The symptoms cause clinically significant distress or impairment in social, occupational, or other important areas of functioning.

D. The symptoms are not due to the direct physiological effects of a substance (e.g., a drug of abuse, a medication) or a general medical condition (e.g., hypothyroidism).

E. The symptoms are not better accounted for by Bereavement, i.e., after the loss of a loved one, the symptoms persist for longer than 2 months or are characterized by marked functional impairment, morbid preoccupation with worthlessness, suicidal ideation, psychotic symptoms, or psychomotor retardation.

Box 1.2 ICD–10 Depressive episode criteria (World Health Organization, 1993. Reprinted by permission.)

F32 Depressive episode

G1. The depressive episode should last for at least 2 weeks.

G2. There have been no hypomanic or manic symptoms sufficient to meet the criteria for hypomanic or manic episode (F30.–) at any time in the individual's life.

G3. *Most commonly used exclusion clause*. The episode is not attributable to psychoactive substance use (F10–F19) or to any organic mental disorder (in the sense of F00–F09).

Somatic syndrome

To qualify for the somatic syndrome, four of the following symptoms should be present:

(1) marked loss of interest or pleasure in activities that are normally pleasurable;

(2) lack of emotional reactions to events or activities that normally produce an emotional response;

(3) waking in the morning 2 hours or more before the usual time;

(4) depression worse in the morning;

(5) objective evidence of marked psychomotor retardation or agitation (remarked on or reported by other people);

(6) marked loss of appetite;

(7) weight loss (5% or more of body weight in the past month);

(8) marked loss of libido.

F32.0 Mild depressive episode

A. The general criteria for depressive episode (F32) must be met.

B. At least two of the following three symptoms must be present:

(1) depressed mood to a degree that is definitely abnormal for the individual, present for most of the day and almost every day, largely uninfluenced by circumstances, and sustained for at least 2 weeks;

(2) loss of interest or pleasure in activities that are normally pleasurable;

(3) decreased energy or increased fatiguability.

C. An additional symptom or symptoms from the following list should be present, to give a total of at least *four*:

(1) loss of confidence or self-esteem;

(2) unreasonable feelings of self-reproach or excessive and inappropriate guilt;

(3) recurrent thoughts of death or suicide, or any suicidal behaviour;

(4) complaints or evidence of diminished ability to think or concentrate, such as indecisiveness or vacillation;

(5) change in psychomotor activity, with agitation or retardation (either subjective or objective);

(6) sleep disturbance of any type;

(7) change in appetite (decrease or increase) with corresponding weight change.

F32.1 Moderate depressive episode

A. The general criteria for depressive episode (F32) must be met.

B. At least two of the three symptoms listed for F32.0, criterion B, must be present.

C. Additional symptoms from F32.0, criterion C, must be present, to give a total of at least *six*.

continued

Box 1.2 *continued*

F32.2 Severe depressive episode without psychotic symptoms

Note: If important symptoms such as agitation or retardation are marked, the patient may be unwilling or unable to describe many symptoms in detail. An overall grading of severe episode may still be justified in such a case.

A. The general criteria for depressive episode (F32) must be met.
B. All three of the symptoms in criterion B, F32.0, must be present.
C. Additional symptoms from F32.0, criterion C, must be present, to give a total of at least *eight*.
D. There must be no hallucinations, delusions, or depressive stupor.

F32.3 Severe depressive episode with psychotic symptoms

A. The general criteria for depressive episode (F32) must be met.
B. The criteria for severe depressive episode without psychotic symptoms (F32.2) must be met with the exception of criterion D.
C. The criteria for schizophrenia (F20.0–F20.3), or schizoaffective disorder, depressive type (F25.1) are not met.
D. Either of the following must be present:
   (1) delusions or hallucinations, other than those listed as typically schizophrenic in criterion G1(1)b, c, and d for F20.0–F20.3 (i.e. delusions other than those that are completely impossible or culturally inappropriate and hallucinations that are not in third person or giving a running commentary); the commonest examples are those with depressive, guilty, hypochondriacal, nihilistic, self-referential, or persecutory content;
   (2) depressive stupor.

F32.8 Other depressive episodes

F32.9 Depressive episode, unspecified

DSM–IV

DSM–IV lists and operationally defines over 300 psychiatric disorders. Each disorder is systematically described in terms of its associated features such as age, gender and culture-related features, incidence risk and predisposing factors. Differential diagnosis is also included. Where relevant, laboratory findings are also described. However, this system is atheoretical and no consideration of causes or treatment is included, nor are controversies surrounding particular diagnoses outlined. It is therefore not a textbook. It also incorporates disorders that are worthy of further scientific examination.

As well as providing detailed criteria for each disorder, DSM–IV is multiaxial in its diagnostic approach, leading to patient evaluation on each of 5 dimensions or axes as follows:

- Axis I   Current mental state diagnosis (definite or provisional)
- Axis II Personality disorder and mental retardation

- Axis III   Any physical condition whether related or not to the psychiatric disorder
- Axis IV   Psychosocial or environmental factors contributing to the disorder
- Axis V   Global Assessment of Functioning (GAF) scale. This is a measure of functioning at a specified time, for example at time of evaluation, highest level of functioning during past 6 months, at time of discharge, etc. This 100-point scale provides a composite measure of psychological, social and occupational functioning. It excludes impairment due to physical or environmental limitations.

In addition, the disorders can be described as mild, moderate or severe, and as possibly being in partial or full remission. Where there is more than one Axis I diagnosis, they are listed in order of the focus of clinical attention. In addition, DSM−IV is hierarchical, so that some diagnoses subsume others, for example if the criteria for schizophrenia and for panic are met, the diagnosis listed is schizophrenia. Organic disorders override psychotic disorders, and these in turn subsume non-psychotic diagnoses. Affective disorders override anxiety disorders. Finally, DSM−IV incorporates, in its appendix, decision trees or algorithms to facilitate diagnosis. A diagnosis can be deemed provisional if there is a strong presumption that the full criteria for the disorder will ultimately be met even though at the time of evaluation it is not possible to make a definitive diagnosis.

ICD−10

This system is now in use throughout Europe and it reflects a significant advance on its predecessor. Many confusing terms such as 'neurotic' are confined to a single category of 'neurotic, stress-related and somatoform disorders', and the older distinction between neurotic and psychotic has been replaced by a classification according to major common themes, for example, mood (affective) disorders (F30−39) and schizophrenia, schizotypal and delusional disorders (F20−29). Childhood disorders have also been incorporated under two broad categories, i.e. disorders of psychological development (F80−89) and behavioural and emotional disorder with onset usually occurring in childhood and adolescence (F90−98). The classification of mental retardation (F70−79) is still rudimentary and is expected to become more comprehensive in subsequent editions.

ICD-10 includes a multiaxial approach although it is somewhat different from DSM in that only 3 axes are recognised and personality disorder is not separated from other mental state disorders. This system also recommends that where multiple Axis I diagnoses coexist (comorbidity) all should be recorded, beginning with the most prominent. Like DSM−IV, ICD−10 is also hierarchical, although diagnostic decision trees are not provided and operational definitions are less rigid than in DSM, allowing for the precedence of clinical judgement.

The axes in ICD−10 are as follow:

- Axis I   Current mental state diagnosis including personality disorder
- Axis II   Disabilities
- Axis III Contextual factors.

Diagnoses may be made with confidence when the diagnostic guidelines are clearly fulfilled. However, if they are only partially met or more information is required the diagnosis may be 'provisional', and the diagnosis is 'tentative' if further information is unlikely to become available. Although guidelines concerning duration are also provided in the criteria, these are not intended as strict requirements and clinicians should use their own judgement when assigning a particular diagnosis if the duration of particular symptoms is slightly shorter or longer than specified.

Interview schedules

In order to carry out epidemiological studies in which diagnoses are standardised, diagnostic interview schedules have been developed that meet the criteria for ICD−10 and DSM−IV diagnoses. In Europe the Schedule for Clinical Assessment in Neuropsychiatry (SCAN) (Wing *et al*, 1990) has evolved from the older Present State Examination (PSE) (Wing *et al*, 1974). SCAN itself is a set of instruments aimed at assessing and classifying psychopathology in adults. The four instruments include PSE−10 (the 10th edition of the Present State Examination), the SCAN glossary, which defines the symptoms; the Item Group Checklist (IGC) for symptoms that can be rated directly (for example from case notes), and the Clinical History Schedule (CHS). This instrument provides diagnoses according to both ICD−10 and DSM−IV criteria. The interview itself is semi-structured, the aim being to encapsulate the clinical interview while minimising its vagaries. There are probe questions with standard wording to elucidate the psychopathological symptoms, defined in the glossary and accompanied by severity ratings. Where there is doubt, the interviewer can proceed to a free-style interview to clarify the feature further and may, if necessary, include the patient's phraseology in questioning to enhance clarity. It is designed for use by psychiatrists or clinical psychologists, thereby utilising clinical interviewing skills in evaluating each symptom. The symptoms ratings, provided they have been identified as defined in the glossary, are then entered into a computer algorithm and a computer diagnosis obtained according to either classification. The role of the interviewer is thus to rate symptoms rather than make diagnoses. SCAN can generate a current diagnosis, a lifetime diagnosis or a representative episode diagnosis. The use of mental health professionals in interviewing with SCAN makes this an expensive method but has the advantage of approximating the 'gold standard' diagnosis achieved by clinical interview.

The DSM−IV equivalent, the Composite International Diagnostic Interview (CIDI) (Robins *et al*, 1989) developed from the Diagnostic Interview Schedule (DIS) (Robins *et al*, 1985), is not a semi-structured interview, but a standardised one, suitable for use with lay interviewers. No clinical judgement is brought to bear in rating the symptoms since questions are asked in a rigid and prescribed manner. The questions are clearly stated to elicit symptoms, followed by questions about frequency, duration and severity. The only judgement the interviewer has to make is whether the respondent understood the question, and if not, it is repeated verbatim. CIDI is available in computer format also and so can be self-administered. As with SCAN, the symptoms are then entered into a computer algorithm for diagnosis according to ICD −10 or DSM−IV. The advantage of this approach is that it is cheaper than using semi-structured interviews, since lay people can be trained in its use. However, the absence of clinical judgement is an obvious disadvantage that has resulted in its validity being questioned. Some recent reviews question the prevalence for some psychiatric disorders obtained using standardised interviews such as CIDI and suggest that the high rates identified in some studies require revision downwards (Regier *et al*, 1998). These mutually different approaches are discussed in detail by Brugha *et al* (1999) and by Wittchen *et al* (1999).

Interviews such as SCAN pay little attention to personality disorder and it is only in the clinical history section that details of diagnoses not covered in PSE−10 are recorded, usually from other sources of information. Likewise CIDI also pays limited attention to personality disorders. Individual categories such as adjustment disorder are only incorporated peripherally in SCAN and not at all in CIDI, thus limiting their usefulness in certain populations where these categories may be common, for example, in primary care and general medical populations respectively.

References

American Psychiatric Association (1952) *Diagnostic and Statistical Manual of Mental Disorders* (1st edn) (DSM−I). Washington, DC: APA.

American Psychiatric Association (1994) *Diagnostic and Statistical Manual of Mental Disorders* (4th edn) (DSM−IV). Washington, DC: APA.

American Psychiatric Association (2000) *Diagnostic and Statistical Manual of Mental Disorders* (4th edn, text revision) (DSM−IV−TR). Washington, DC: APA.

Brugha, T. S., Bebbington, P. E. & Jenkins, R. (1999) A difference that matters: comparisons of structured and semi-structured psychiatric diagnostic interviews in the general population. *Psychological Medicine*, **29**, 1013−1020.

Jaspers, K. (1962) *General Psychopathology* (7th edn), (trans. J. Hoenig & M. W. Hamilton). Manchester: Manchester University Press.

Regier, D. A., Kaelber, C. T., Rae, D. S., *et al* (1998) Limitations of diagnostic criteria and assessment instruments for mental disorders. Implications for research and policy. *Archives of General Psychiatry*, **55**, 105−115.

Robins, L. N., Helzer, J. E., Orvaschel, H., *et al* (1985) The Diagnostic Interview Schedule. In *Epidemiologic Field Methods in Psychiatry: The NIMH Epidemiologic Catchment Area Program* (eds W. W. Eaton & L. G. Kessler), pp. 143−170. Orlando, Academic Press.

Robins, L. N., Wing, J., Wittchen, H. U., *et al* (1989) The Composite International Diagnostic Interview: An epidemiologic instrument suitable for use in conjunction with different diagnostic systems and in different cultures. *Archives of General Psychiatry*, **45**, 1069–1077.

Schneider, K. (1959) *Clinical Psychopathology* (5th edn), (trans. M. W. Hamilton). New York: Grune & Stratton.

Wing, J. K., Cooper, J. & Sartorius, N. (1974) *Measurement and Classification of Psychiatric Symptoms*. New York: Cambridge University Press.

Wing, J. K., Babor, T., Brugha, T., *et al* (1990) SCAN: Schedules for Clinical Assessment in Neuropsychiatry. *Archives of General Psychiatry*, **47**, 589–593.

Wittchen, H. -U., Ustun, T. B. & Kessler, R. C. (1999) Diagnosing mental disorders in the community. A difference that matters? *Psychological Medicine*, **29**, 1021–1027.

World Health Organization (1992) *The ICD–10 Classification of Mental and Behavioural Disorders. Clinical Descriptions and Diagnostic Guidelines* (10th edn). Geneva: WHO.

World Health Organization (1993) *The ICD–10 Classification of Mental and Behavioural Disorders. Diagnostic Criteria for Research* (10th edn). Geneva: WHO.

World Health Organization (1996) *ICD–10 Diagnostic and Management Guidelines for Mental Disorders in Primary Care*. Geneva: WHO.

CHAPTER 2

Disorders of perception

Disorders of perception can be divided into sensory distortions and sensory deceptions. In distortions there is a constant real perceptual object, which is perceived in a distorted way, while in sensory deceptions a new perception occurs that may or may not be in response to an external stimulus.

Sensory distortions

These are changes in perception that are the result of a change in the intensity and quality of the stimulus or the spatial form of the perception.

Changes in intensity (hyper- or hypo-aesthesia)

Increased intensity of sensations (hyperaesthesia) may be the result of intense emotions or a lowering of the physiological threshold. Thus a person may see roof tiles as a brilliant flaming red or hear the noise of a door closing like a clap of thunder. Anxiety and depressive disorders as well as hangover from alcohol and migraine are all associated with increased sensitivity to noise (hyperacusis) so that even day-to-day noises such as washing crockery are magnified to the point of discomfort. Those who are hypomanic, suffering an epileptic aura or under the influence of lysergic acid diethylamide (LSD) may see colours as very bright and intense, but this can also be a feature of intense normal emotions such as religious fervour or the unsurpassed happiness of being in love.

Hypoacusis occurs in delirium, where the threshold for all sensations is raised. The defect of attention found in delirium further reduces sensory acuity. This highlights the importance of speaking to the delirious patient more slowly and louder than usual. Hypoacusis is also a feature of other disorders associated with attentional deficits such as depression and attention-deficit disorder. Visual and gustatory sensations may also be lowered in depression, for example, everything is black or all foods taste the same.

Changes in quality

It is mainly visual perceptions that are affected by this, brought about by toxic substances. Colouring of yellow, green and red have been named xanthopsia, chloropsia and erythropsia. These are mainly the result of drugs (for example, santonin, poisoning with mescaline or digitalis) used in the past to treat various disorders. The qualitative change most associated with drugs now is the metallic taste associated with the use of lithium, although this is not a hallucination but a true change in gustation. In derealisation everything appears unreal and strange, while in mania objects look perfect and beautiful.

Changes in spatial form (dysmegalopsia)

This refers to a change in the perceived shape of an object. Micropsia is a visual disorder in which the patient sees objects as smaller than they really are. The opposite kind of visual experience is known as macropsia or megalopsia. This definition of micropsia includes the experience of the retreat of objects into the distance without any change in size although some authors call this porropsia. The terms macropsia and micropsia have also been used to describe the changes of size in dreams and hallucinations (Lilliputian hallucinations). Some authors reserve the term dysmegalopsia to describe objects that are perceived to be larger (or smaller) on one side than the other (Sims, 2003), while others use the term generically to describe any change in perceived size (Hamilton, 1974). Others use the term metamorphosia rather than dysmegalopsia to describe objects that are irregular in shape.

Dysmegalopsia can result from retinal disease, disorders of accommodation and convergence but most commonly from temporal and parietal lobe lesions. Rarely, it can be associated with schizophrenia. In oedema of the retina visual elements are separated so that the image falls on what is functionally a smaller part of the retina than usual. This gives rise to micropsia. Scarring of the retina with retraction naturally produces macropsia, but as the distortion produced by scarring is usually irregular, metamorphopsia is more likely to result.

Complete paralysis of accommodation or overactivity of accommodation during near vision is likely to cause macropsia, while partial paralysis of accommodation will lead to the experience during near vision that the object is very near, i.e. micropsia will occur. If accommodation is normal but convergence is weakened, macropsia occurs and vice versa.

Despite the fact that disorders of accommodation and convergence can cause dysmegalopsia, it is not common to meet cases in which the visual disorder is the result of a failure of these peripheral mechanisms. Occasionally dysmegalopsia may occur in poisoning with atropine or hyoscine. Although hypoxia and rapid acceleration of the body can disturb accommodation and convergence, dysmegalopsia is rare among high-altitude pilots. Sometimes the nerves controlling accommodation are affected by conditions such as chronic arachnoiditis and this may give rise to dysmegalopsia. However, it is more common in central lesions, mainly those affecting the posterior temporal lobe, and macropsia, micropsia or irregular distortions may occur either during the aura or in the course of the fit itself.

Distortions of the experience of time

From the psychopathological point of view there are two varieties of time: physical and personal, the latter being determined by personal judgement of the passage of time. It is the latter that is affected by psychiatric disorders. We are all aware of the influence of mood on the passage of time, so that when we are happy 'time flies', and when we are sad it passes more slowly. In severe depression the patient may feel that time passes very slowly and even stands still. Slowing down of time is most marked in those with psychotic depressive symptoms. By contrast the manic patient feels that time speeds by and that the days are not long enough to do everything. Some patients with schizophrenia believe that time moves in fits and starts, and may have a delusional elaboration that clocks are being interfered with.

In acute organic states, disorders of personal time are shown in temporal disorientation and in milder forms there may be an overestimation of the progress of time. Some patients with temporal lobe lesions may complain that time either passes slowly or quickly.

In recent years there is some evidence to suggest that patients with schizophrenia have abnormalities of time judgement, estimating intervals to be less than they are. Age disorientation is another feature present in patients with chronic schizophrenia, noted even in the absence of any other features of confusion (Tapp *et al*, 1993; Manschreck *et al*, 2000).

Sensory deceptions

These can be divided into illusions, which are misinterpretations of stimuli arising from an external object, and hallucinations, which are perceptions without an adequate external stimulus.

Illusions

In illusions, stimuli from a perceived object are combined with a mental image to produce a false perception. It is unfortunate that the word 'illusion' is also used for perceptions that do not agree with the physical stimuli, such as the Muller-Lyer illusion in which two lines of equal length can be made to appear unequal depending on the direction of the arrowheads at the end of each respectively. Illusions in themselves are not indicative of psychopathology since they can occur in the absence of psychiatric disorder, for example the person walking along a dark road may misinterpret innocuous shadows as threatening attackers. Illusions can occur in delirium when the perceptual threshold is raised and an anxious and bewildered patient misinterprets stimuli. While visual illusions are the most common, they can occur in any modality. For example, auditory illusions may occur when a person hears words in a conversation that resemble their own name and they believe they are being talked about. At times it is difficult to be certain that the patient is describing an illusion or whether he is actually hearing hallucinatory voices talking about him and attributing them to real people in his environment.

The classic psychiatrists described fantastic illusions in which patients saw extraordinary modifications to their environment. One had a patient who looked in the mirror and instead of seeing his own head saw that of a pig. Fish (1974) had a patient who insisted that during an interview he saw the psychiatrist's head change into that of a rabbit. This patient was given to exaggeration and confabulation. He would also invent non-existent puppies and tell other patients not to tread on them. However, fantastic illusions belong more in the worlds of fiction than in the realm of psychiatry (Hamilton, 1974).

Three types of illusion are described (Sims, 2003) as follows:

- Completion illusions: these depend on inattention such as misreading words in newspapers or missing misprints because we read the word as if it were complete. Alternatively, if we see faded letters we may misread the word on the basis of our previous experience, our interests etc., for example, to the person with an interest in reading, the word '–ook' might be misread as 'book' even though the faded letter was an 'l'.

- Affect illusions: these arise in the context of a particular mood state. For example, a bereaved person may momentarily believe they 'see' the deceased person, or the delirious person in a perplexed and bewildered state may perceive the innocent gestures of others as threatening. In severe depression when delusions of guilt are present the person, believing that he is wicked, may also say that he hears people talking about killing him when he is in the company of others. In these circumstances it is difficult to know if he is experiencing illusions or hearing hallucinatory voices talking about him and attributing them to those around him.

- Pareidolia: this is an interesting type of illusion, in which vivid illusions occur without the patient making any effort. These illusions are the result of excessive fantasy thinking and a vivid visual imagery. They cannot therefore be explained as the result of affect or mind-set, so that they differ from the ordinary illusion. Pareidolias occur when the subject sees vivid pictures in fire or in clouds, without any conscious effort on his part and sometimes even against his will.

Illusions have to be distinguished from intellectual misunderstanding and the latter is usually obvious. Thus when someone says that a piece of rock is a precious stone this may be a misunderstanding based on lack of knowledge. The distinction between an illusion and a functional hallucination (see p. 26) may be more difficult. Both occur in response to an environmental stimulus but in a functional hallucination both the stimulus and the hallucination are perceived by the patient simultaneously, and can be identified as separate and not as a transformation of the stimulus. This contrasts with an illusion in which the stimulus from the environment changes but forms an essential and integral part of the new perception.

Trailing phenomena, although not strictly illusions, are perceptual abnormalities in which moving objects are seen as a series of discreet and discontinuous images. They are associated with hallucinogenic drugs.

Hallucinations

Definitions

The definition of a hallucination as 'a perception without an object' has the advantage of being simple and to the point but is does not quite cover functional hallucinations. To cover these and to exclude dreams Jaspers suggested the following definition 'a false perception which is not a sensory distortion or a misinterpretation, but which occurs at the same time as real perceptions'. SCAN (World Health Organization, 1998) defines hallucinations as 'false perceptions'.

What distinguishes hallucinations from true perceptions is that they come from 'within', although the subject reacts to them as if they were true perceptions coming from 'without'. This distinguishes them from vivid mental images that also come from within but are recognised as such. As with all abnormal mental phenomena, it is not possible to make an absolute distinction as the individual with eidetic imagery will examine his images as if they were external objects and some patients have sufficient insight to recognise that their hallucinations are not truly objective.

A great deal of discussion has raged about the concept of the 'pseudo-hallucination'. Most of the statements are derived from the work of Jaspers (1962), who, first of all, distinguished between true perceptions and mental images. Perceptions are substantial; appear in objective space; are clearly delineated, constant and independent of the will; and their sensory elements are full and fresh. Mental images are incomplete; are not clearly delineated; are dependent on the will; exist in subjective space; are inconstant and have to be recreated. Pseudo-hallucinations are a type of mental image that, although clear and vivid, lack the substantiality of perceptions; they are seen in full consciousness, known to be not real perceptions and are located not in objective space but in subjective space (for example, inside the head). Like true hallucinations they are involuntary. In his book *General Psychopathology* Jaspers (1962) gives two examples, one of a patient who had taken opium, making it unlikely therefore that the pseudo-hallucination appeared in clear consciousness. The second concerned a patient with a chronic psychotic illness who himself distinguished between hallucinatory voices in objective space and voices which he heard inwardly (pseudo-hallucinations). Pseudo-hallucinations can be identified in the auditory, tactile or visual modalities.

The confusion over the meaning of 'pseudo-hallucination' stems from two different approaches to definition; one based on insight (Hare, 1973) and the other, as exemplified by Jaspers (1962), based on whether the image lies in inner or outer perceptual space. Jaspers believed that pseudo-hallucinations are variants of fantasy/mental imagery and, thus not carrying the same diagnostic implications, are true hallucinations. Hare argued that since insight often fluctuates and at times is partial, it was more profitable to think in terms of degree of insight. This, however, renders the concept of pseudo-hallucinations largely superfluous. SCAN (World Health Organization, 1998) does not use the term pseudo-hallucination, but does have an item for rating insight and for whether the experience occurs inside or outside the head.

Jaspers insisted that there is no gradual transition between true and pseudo-hallucinations, but Fish, in a previous edition of this book (Hamilton, 1974) disagreed, citing an example of non-substantial hallucinations experienced in outer objective space; patients with substantial hallucinations also experienced these in outer objective space but they recognised these as the result of their active vivid imagination. Thus, Fish argued, there is a continuum from pseudo-hallucinations to hallucinations. This is confirmed by the work of Leff (1968) on sensory deprivation and perception. He found that subjects could not always distinguish between images and hallucinations and concluded that the perceptual experiences of normal people under conditions of sensory deprivation overlap considerably with those of psychiatric patients.

The importance of pseudo-hallucinations is that their presence does not necessarily indicate psychopathology, unlike true hallucinations, which are indicative of serious mental illness. Although such a comment is found in many textbooks of psychiatry, its veracity must surely rest with the definition that is adopted, since, as Hare argues, if insight is the criterion and this fluctuates during illness, the meaning and relevance of pseudo-hallucinations becomes redundant.

Causes

Hallucinations can be the result of intense emotions or psychiatric disorder, suggestion, disorders of sense organs, sensory deprivation and disorders of the central nervous system.

Emotion

Very depressed patients with delusions of guilt may hear voices reproaching them. These are not the continuous voices of paranoid schizophrenia or organic hallucinosis but tend to be disjointed or fragmentary, uttering single words or short phrases such as 'rotter', 'kill yourself', etc. The occurrence of continuous persistent hallucinatory voices in severe depression should arouse the suspicion of schizophrenia or some intercurrent physical disease. On the other hand the hallucinations that occur in schizophrenia are often of a persecutory nature and may consist of voices giving a commentary on the person's actions and discussing him in a hostile manner.

Suggestion

Several experimenters have shown that normal subjects can be persuaded to hallucinate. When asked to walk down a dimly lit corridor and stop when they saw a faint light over the door at the end, most subjects stopped walking at some time during the study saying they could see a light even though none was switched on. Similarly subjects can be persuaded to hallucinate visually or auditorily, either by hypnosis or by brief task-motivating instructions. This latter technique consists in asking the subject to try to hallucinate a tune or an animal and then telling him that much more must be done as most people can hallucinate if they try hard enough. A group in whom suggestion was believed to be relevant to the genesis of hallucinations (Hamilton, 1974) were those with a diagnosis of the so-called 'hysterical psychosis'. The hallucinations, visual in nature, were said to conform to the patient's fantasies and cultural background. However, this diagnosis is no longer specifically mentioned, either as a specific category or an inclusion category, in either ICD–10 or DSM–IV and so is only of historical interest. The belief that Ganser syndrome is psychogenic in origin (Ungvari & Mullen, 1997) opens the possibility of the role of suggestion in the genesis of the hallucinations in this condition, although others dispute this and regard it as an organic condition (Latcham et al, 1978). The syndrome is now recognised to occur in a variety of psychiatric disorders, including schizophrenia, dissociative disorder, malingering, organic states, etc.

Disorders of a peripheral sense organ

Hallucinatory voices may occur in ear disease and visual hallucinations in diseases of the eye, but often there is some disorder of the central nervous system as well. For example, a woman aged 66 suffered from glaucoma and then began to have continuous visual hallucinations. At the time she showed evidence of atherosclerotic dementia and had a focus of abnormal activity in the left posterior temporal lobe. Charles Bonnet syndrome (phantom visual images) is a condition in which complex visual hallucinations occur in the absence of any psychopathology and in clear consciousness. It is associated with either central or peripheral reduction in vision and not surprisingly is most common in the elderly but can occur in younger people also. The hallucinatory episodes are of variable duration and can last for years. The images may be static or in motion and the importance of this diagnosis is as a differential from psychopathological causes of hallucinations. Peripheral lesions of sense organs may play a part in hallucinations in organic states and it has been shown that negative scotomota are to be found in patients with alcohol misuse.

Sensory deprivation

If all incoming stimuli are reduced to a minimum in a normal subject, they will begin to hallucinate after a few hours. These hallucinations are usually changing visual hallucinations and repetitive words and phrases. It has been suggested that the sensory isolation produced by deafness may cause paranoid disorders in the deaf (Cooper, 1976). Similarly, sensory deprivation due to the use of protective patches may contribute to the delirium that follows cataract surgery, along with mild cognitive deficits due to ageing. There is an interesting case on record of a patient who had 'black patch disease' after an operation and was frightened by the prospect of another operation on her other eye a few years later. She was reassured by a psychiatrist, who saw her before and immediately afterwards and promised to see her whenever requested during the post-operative period. After the second operation she had no hallucinations of any kind.

Disorders of the central nervous system
Lesions of the diencephalons and the cortex can produce hallucinations that are usually visual but can be auditory.

Hypnagogic and hypnopompic hallucinations are special kinds of organic hallucination (see below).

Hallucinations of individual senses
Before deciding that a patient is hallucinated, the possibility of other explanations must be considered; these are not necessarily of pathological significance. The differential diagnosis of hallucinations includes illusions, pseudo-hallucinations, hypnagogic and hypnopompic images, vivid imagery and normal perceptions. The possibility that the experience is a delusion without a hallucination, although described as if it were a perceptual abnormality, must also be considered, for example 'people talk about me' (when in fact the patient does not hear others talking but believes they are doing so).

Hearing (auditory)
Hallucinatory voices were called 'phonemes' by Wernicke in 1900, although this term, a technical one derived from linguistics, is rarely used now. Auditory hallucination may be elementary and unformed, and experienced as simple noises, bells, undifferentiated whispers or voices. Elementary auditory hallucinations can occur in organic states and noises, partly organised as music or completely organised as hallucinatory voices, in schizophrenia. In the latter they may form a part of the basis for the patient's delusion that they are the victim of persecution or that their thoughts or actions are being controlled. 'Voices' are characteristic of schizophrenia and can occur at any stage of the illness. As well as occurring in organic states, such as delirium or dementia, they can occasionally occur in severe depression but they are usually less well formed than those described in schizophrenia.

Hallucinatory voices vary in quality, ranging from those that are quite clear and can be ascribed to specific individuals to those that are vague and which the patient cannot describe with any clarity. Patients are often undisturbed by their inability to describe the direction from which the voices come or the sex of the person speaking. This is quite unlike the experience of the healthy individual. The voices sometimes give instructions to the patient, who may or may not act upon them; these are termed 'imperative hallucinations'. In some cases the voices speak about the person in the third person and may give a running commentary on their actions. These are among Schneider's first-rank symptoms, and although this was one thought to be diagnostic of schizophrenia, this is no longer the case since these symptoms have also been described in mania (Gonzalez-Pinto *et al*, 2003). Auditory hallucinations may be abusive, neutral or even helpful in tone. At times they may speak incomprehensible nonsense or neologisms.

The effect of the voices on the patient's behaviour is variable. A number of patients (becoming fewer in number with advances in treatment) have continuous hallucinations that do not trouble them. For others the persistence of the hallucinations cuts across all activities so that the patient is seen to be listening and even replying to them at times. Sometimes activity may diminish due to preoccupation with the hallucinations.

One type of auditory hallucination is hearing one's own thoughts spoken aloud and is also one of Schneider's first-rank symptoms. Known in German as *Gedankenlautwerden*, it describes hearing one's thoughts spoken just before or at the same time as they are occurring. *Echo de la pensée* (French) is the phenomenon of hearing them spoken after the thoughts have occurred. Probably the best English term would be 'thought echo' or the alternative and more cumbersome 'thought sonorisation'. Of note, SCAN classifies thought echo as a disorder of thought (World Health Organization, 1998) rather than as a hallucinatory experience. The patient may also complain that their thoughts are no longer private but are accessible to others. This is known as thought broadcasting or thought diffusion (also a first-rank symptom) and is best classified as a disorder of thought rather than a hallucinatory experience, since there is no necessary implication that thoughts must first be heard. However, there are different definitions of this phenomenon, some of which specify that the thoughts must first be audible, so that *Gedankenlautwerden/echo de la pensee* are prerequisites to thought broadcast (Pawar & Spence, 2003).

Patients explain the origin of the voices in different ways. They may insist that the voices are the result of witchcraft, telepathy, radio, television, and so on. Sometimes they claim that the voices come from within their bodies such as their arms, legs, stomach, etc. For example, one patient heard the voices of two nurses and the Crown Prince of Germany coming from her chest. Some patients hallucinate speech movements and hear speech that comes from their own throat but has no connection with their thinking. One patient complained bitterly of her 'talky-talky tongue' because she was continuously auditorily hallucinated and felt speech movements in her tongue. Thus she had both auditory and possibly somatic hallucinations. However, it has been shown that sub-vocal speech movements occur in healthy subjects when they are thinking or reading silently, and it has also been demonstrated that patients hearing voices have slight movements of the lips, tongue and laryngeal muscles and that there is an increase in the action potentials in the laryngeal muscles. It is perhaps surprising that more patients do not complain of voices coming from their throat or tongue.

A few patients deny hearing voices but assert that people are talking about them. Careful investigation of the content and nature of the things that others are alleged to have said may show that the patient has continuous hallucinations and attributes them to real people in the vicinity. As these are often abusive the patient may attack those whom they believe are responsible. A good example of this was a Greek woman who had been a patient in a long-stay ward for many years. She always denied hearing voices but from time to time would make unprovoked attacks on fellow patients. One day she was asked if she would like some Greek newspapers or visits from someone who spoke Greek. She said that this was not necessary because everybody in the hospital spoke Greek. It became obvious that she heard continuous voices in Greek that she attributed to real people, and that her seemingly motiveless attacks were prompted by this. This clearly represented a delusional elaboration of a hallucinatory experience.

Vision

These may be elementary in the form of flashes of light, partly organised in the form of patterns, or completely organised in the form of visions of people, objects or animals. Figures of living things and inanimate objects may appear against the normally perceived environment or scenic hallucinations can occur in which whole scenes are hallucinated rather like a cinema film.

All varieties of visual hallucination are found in acute organic states but small animals and insects are most often hallucinated in delirium. One patient in delirium tremens described mice carrying suitcases on their backs as they boarded a flight to Lourdes. These hallucinations are usually associated with fear and terror. Patients with delirium tremens are extremely suggestible so that one may be able to persuade the patient to read a blank sheet of paper; one investigator produced a disc of light by pressing on the patient's eyeball and persuaded him that he could see a dog. Scenic hallucinations are common in psychiatric disorders associated with epilepsy and these patients may also have visions of fire and religious scenes such as the Crucifixion.

Often, visual hallucinations are isolated and do not have any accompanying voices. Sometimes, however, visual and auditory hallucinations co-occur to form a coherent whole. Patients with temporal-lobe epilepsy may have combined auditory and visual hallucinations and some patients with schizophrenia of late onset (especially when the illness is protracted) may see and hear people being tortured, murdered and mutilated.

In some patients, micropsia affects visual hallucinations so that they see tiny people or objects, so-called Lilliputian hallucinations. Unlike the usual organic visual hallucinations, these are accompanied by pleasure and amusement. For example, one patient with delirium tremens was very pleased when she saw a tiny German band playing on her counterpane. When these occur in delirium tremens the patient exhibits a combination of child-like pleasure and terror.

Visual hallucinations are more common in acute organic states with clouding of consciousness than in functional psychosis. The disturbance of consciousness makes it difficult for the patient to distinguish between mental images and perceptions, although this is sometimes possible. Visual hallucinations are extremely rare in schizophrenia, so much so that they should raise a doubt about the diagnosis. Some patients with schizophrenia describe visions and these appear to be pseudo-hallucinations, but on occasion others will insist that their hallucinations are substantial.

Occasionally visual hallucinations occur in the absence of any psychopathology or brain disease and Charles Bonnet syndrome must then be considered as the most likely differential diagnosis.

Smell (olfactory)

Hallucinations of odour can occur in schizophrenia and organic states and, uncommonly, in depressive psychosis. It may be difficult to be sure if there is a hallucination or an illusion. There may also be a problem distinguishing olfactory hallucination from delusion since there are some people who insist that they emit a smell. It is important to ascertain if they actually smell this odour, since many seem to base their belief on the behaviour of other people who, they say, wrinkle their noses or make reference to the smell. Some patients with schizophrenia claim that they smell gas and that their enemies are poisoning them by pumping gas into the room. Episodes of temporal lobe disturbance are often ushered in by an aura involving an unpleasant odour such as burning paint or rubber. At times, the hallucination may occur without any fit so that the patient then complains of a strange smell in the house. For example one patient with a temporal lobe focus had no fits but, from time to time, would complain of a smell of stale cabbage water in the house and would turn the house upside down trying to locate the offending object. Sometimes the smell may be pleasant, for example when some religious people can smell roses around certain saints; this is known as the Padre Pio phenomenon.

Taste (gustatory)

Hallucinations of taste occur in schizophrenia and acute organic states but it is not always easy to know whether the patient actually tastes something odd or if it is a delusional explanation of the effect of feeling strangely changed. Depressed patients often describe a loss of taste or state that all food tastes the same.

Touch (tactile)

This may take the form of small animals crawling over the body, so-called formication. This is not uncommon in acute organic states. In cocaine psychosis this type of hallucination commonly occurs together with delusions of persecution and is known as the 'cocaine bug'. Some patients experience the feeling of cold winds blowing on them, sensations of heat, electrical shocks and sexual sensations, and the patient is convinced that these are produced by outside agencies. In the absence of coarse brain disease, the most likely diagnosis is schizophrenia. Indeed, Sims (2003) points out that there is almost always a concomitant delusional elaboration of tactile hallucinatory experiences. Sexual hallucinations can occur in both acute and chronic schizophrenia, for example, one patient complained that she could feel the penis of her son's employer in her vagina no matter what she did and although she could not see the man she was certain of this.

Sims (2003) classifies tactile hallucinations into three main types: superficial, kinaestethic and visceral (see below). Sims further divides superficial hallucinations, which affect the skin, into four types: thermic (e.g. a cold wind blowing across the face), haptic (e.g. feeling a hand brushing against the skin), hygric (e.g. feeling fluid such as water running from the head into the stomach) and paraestethic (pins and needles), although the latter most often have an organic origin. Kinaestethic hallucinations affect the muscles and joints and the patient feels that their limbs are being twisted, pulled or moved. They occur in schizophrenia, where they can be distinguished from delusions of passivity by the presence of definite sensations. Vestibular sensations such as sinking in the bed or flying through the air can also be hallucinated and are best regarded as a variant of kinaestethic hallucinations and occur in organic states, most commonly delirium tremens. Kinaestethic or vestibular perceptions occur in organic states such as alcohol intoxication and during benzodiazepine withdrawal and may also occur in the absence of any abnormality, for example after a week's sailing an undulating feeling may persist for a few days.

Pain and deep sensation

These are termed visceral hallucinations by Sims (2003). Some patients with chronic schizophrenia may complain of twisting and tearing pains. These may be very bizarre when the patient complains that his organs are being torn out or the flesh ripped away from his body. For example, a patient described sensations in his brain as layers of tissue were being peeled off so as to bring to completion the battle between good and evil.

An interesting and unusual variety of hallucinosis is delusional zoopathy. This may take the form of a delusional belief that there is an animal crawling about in the body. There is also a hallucinatory component since the patient feels it (hallucination) and can describe it in detail. In some cases this is associated with an organic disorder, as in the patient who said he was infested with an animal several centimetres long that he could feel in his stomach. He eventually died and at post mortem was found to have a tumour invading the thalamus.

The sense of 'presence'

It is difficult to classify an abnormal sense of presence because, although it is not strictly a sense deception, it cannot be regarded as a delusion either.

Most normal people have from time to time the sense that someone is present when they are alone, on a dark street or climbing a dimly lit staircase. Often the feeling is that there is somebody behind them. Usually this is dismissed as imagination but nevertheless they look behind them to be certain. However, sometimes there is the feeling that someone is present, whom they cannot see, and may or may not be able to name. For example, Saint Teresa of Avila wrote,

'One day when I was at prayer – it was the feast-day of the glorious Saint Peter – I saw Christ at my side – or, to put it better, I was conscious of Him, for I saw nothing with the eyes of the body or the eyes of the soul. He seemed quite close to me, and I saw that it was He'.

She says a little later,

'But I felt most clearly that he was all the time on my right, and was a witness of everything that I was doing'.

This experience was probably the result of lack of sleep, hunger and religious enthusiasm. It may also have been a metaphorical way of describing closeness to God/Christ. One patient described a presence over her right shoulder that followed her from room to room and even though she knew that there was nobody there, the feeling was intense and distressing, so much so that at times she hid under the bedclothes to escape.

The sense of a presence can occur in healthy people as well as in organic states, schizophrenia or hysteria and the patient described above also had a diagnosis of borderline personality disorder.

Hallucinatory syndromes

Hallucinatory syndromes, also termed hallucinosis, refer to those disorders in which there are persistent hallucinations in any sensory modality in the absence of other psychotic features. The main hallucinatory syndromes that are identified are:

- alcoholic hallucinosis; these hallucinations are usually auditory and occur during periods of relative abstinence. They may be threatening or reproachful, although some patients report benign voices. Sensorium is clear and hallucinations rarely persist longer than 1 week and are associated with long-standing alcohol misuse
- organic hallucinosis; these are present in 20–30% of patients with dementia, especially of the Alzheimer type, and are most commonly auditory or visual. There is also disorientation and memory is impaired.

Special kinds of hallucination

Functional hallucinations

An auditory stimulus causes a hallucination but the stimulus is experienced as well as the hallucination. In other words the hallucination requires the presence of another real sensation. For example, a patient with schizophrenia first heard the voice of God as her clock ticked; later she heard voices coming from the running tap and voices coming from the chirruping of the birds.

So both the noises and the voices were audible. Patients can distinguish both features from each other and crucially, the hallucination does not occur without the stimulus. Some patients who discover that noises induce hallucinatory voices put plugs in their ears to reduce the intensity of the stimulus and hence the hallucinations. One patient recently described that she saw the mouths of her collection of dolls moving. The perception of dolls was necessary to produce the hallucination but the movement of their mouths was distinct and separate and did not represent a transformation of that perception, thus making this a functional hallucination rather than an illusion. Functional hallucinations are not uncommon in chronic schizophrenia and they may be mistaken for illusions.

Reflex hallucinations
Synaesthesia is the experience of a stimulus in one sense modality producing a sensory experience in another. For example, the feeling of cold in one's spine on hearing a fingernail scratch a blackboard. One patient described hearing his own reflection and said that when attempting to carry out some action he could hear himself doing so. Although rare, synaesthesia can occur under the influence of hallucinogenic drugs such as LSD or mescaline when the subject might describe feeling, tasting and hearing flowers simultaneously. Reflex hallucinations are a morbid form of synaesthesia. In a reflex hallucination a stimulus in one sensory field produces a hallucination in another. For example, a patient felt a pain in her head (somatic hallucination) when she heard other people sneeze (the stimulus) and was convinced that sneezing caused the pain.

Extracampine hallucinations
The patient has a hallucination that is outside the limits of the sensory field. For example, a patient sees somebody standing behind them when they are looking straight ahead or hear voices talking in London when they are in Liverpool. These hallucinations can occur in healthy people as hypnagogic hallucinations but also in schizophrenia or organic conditions, including epilepsy.

Autoscopy or phantom mirror-image
Autoscopy, also called phantom mirror-image, is the experience of seeing oneself and knowing that it is oneself. It is not just a visual hallucination because kinaestethic and somatic sensation must also be present to give the subject the impression that the hallucination is oneself. This symptom can occur in healthy subjects when they are emotionally upset or when exhausted. In these cases there is some change in the state of consciousness. Occasionally autoscopy is a hysterical symptom. Occasionally patients with schizophrenia have autoscopic hallucinations but they are more common in acute and sub-acute delirious states. The organic states most associated with autoscopy are epilepsy, focal lesions affecting the parieto−occipital region and toxic infective states whose effect is greatest in the basal regions of the brain. The fact that autoscopy is often associated with disorders of

the parietal lobe due to cerebrovascular disorders or severe infectious diseases accounts for the German folklore belief that when someone sees their double or Doppelganger it indicates that they are about to die. Sometimes these may be pseudo-hallucinations occurring in internal space and described by the patient as being 'in the mind's eye'.

A few patients suffering from organic states look in the mirror and see no image, known as negative autoscopy. Some psychiatrists describe internal autoscopy in which the subject sees their own internal organs, although this is rare. The description of the internal organs is that which would be expected from a layperson, with a crude knowledge of anatomy.

Hypnagogic and hypnopompic hallucinations

First mentioned by Aristotle, these hallucinations occur when the subject is falling asleep or waking up respectively. It has been suggested that hypnopompic hallucinations are often hypnagogic experiences that occur in the morning when the subject is waking and dosing-off again, so that they actually happen when the subject is falling asleep. The term 'hypnopompic' should be reserved for those hallucinatory experiences that persist from sleep when the eyes are open. Hypnagogic hallucinations occur during drowsiness, are discontinuous, appear to force themselves on the subject and do not form part of an experience in which the subject participates as they do in a dream. They are about three times more common (described by 37% of the adult population) than hypnopompic hallucinations, although the latter are a better indicator of narcolepsy. The subject believes that the hallucination has woken them up (for example, hearing the telephone ring even though it has not) and although the auditory modality is the most common it can also be visual, kinaestethic or tactile and is sudden in occurrence. Subjects describing hypnagogic hallucinations often assert that they are fully awake. This is not so and electroencephalogram (EEG) records show that there is a low of alpha rhythm at the time of the hallucination.

Hypnagogic visual hallucinations may be geometrical designs, abstract shapes, faces, figures or scenes from nature. Auditory hallucinations may be animal noises, music or voices. One of the most common is that of hearing one's name called or a voice saying a sentence or phrase that has no discoverable meaning. In a subject deprived of sleep a hypnagogic state may occur, in which case there are hallucinatory voices, visual hallucinations, ideas of reference and no insight into the morbid phenomena. It resolves once the subject has a good sleep.

The importance of hypnagogic and hypnopompic phenomena is to recognise that they are not indicative of any psychopathology even though they are true hallucinatory experiences (Ohayon et al, 1996). They also occur in narcolepsy.

Organic hallucinations

Organic hallucinations can occur in any sensory modality and they may occur in a variety of neurological and psychiatric disorders. The focus in this section will be on the psychiatric causes.

Organic visual hallucinations occur in eye disorders as well as in disorders of the central nervous system and lesions of the optic tract. Complex scenic hallucinations occur in temporal lobe lesions. Charles Bonnet syndrome consists of visual hallucinations in the absence of any other psychopathology, although impaired vision is present. All the dementias as well as delirium and substance abuse are associated with visual hallucinations.

The phantom limb is the most common organic somatic hallucination of psychiatric origin. In this case the patient feels that they have a limb from which in fact they are not receiving any sensations either because it has been amputated or because the sensory pathways from it have been destroyed. In rare cases with thalamo−parietal lesions the patient describes a third limb. In most phantom limbs the phenomenon is produced by peripheral and central disorders. Phantom limb occurs in about 95% of all amputations after the age of 6 years. Occasionally a phantom limb develops after a lesion of the peripheral nerve or the medulla or spinal cord. The phantom limb does not necessarily correspond to the previous image of the limb in that it may be shorter or consist only of the distal portion so that the phantom hand arises from the shoulder. If there is clouding of consciousness, the patient may be deluded that the limb is real. Equivalent perceptions of phantom organs may also occur after other surgical procedures such as mastectomy, enucleation of the eye, removal of the larynx or the construction of a colostomy. The person is aware of the existence of the organ or limb and describes pain or paraesthesia in the space occupied by the phantom organ and this persists in a minority of patients. When the experience is related to a limb the perception shrinks over time, with distal parts disappearing more quickly than those that are proximal. Lesions of the parietal lobe can also produce somatic hallucinations with distortion or splitting-off of body parts.

Lesions of the temporal lobe are associated with multi-sensory hallucinations but they do not include somatic hallucinations, which is to be expected because the somatic sensory area is separated from the temporal lobe by the Sylvian fissure.

The patient's attitude to hallucinations

In organic hallucinations the patient is usually terrified by the visual hallucinations and may try desperately to get away from them. Most delirious patients feel threatened and are generally suspicious. The combination of the persecuted attitude and the visual hallucinations may lead to resistance to all nursing care and to impulsive attempts to escape from the threatening situation, so that they may jump out of windows and jeopardise their lives. The exception is Lilliputian hallucinations, which are usually regarded with amusement by the patient and may be watched with delight.

Patients with depression often hear disjointed voices abusing them or telling them to kill themselves. They are not terrified by the voices, as they believe they are wicked and deserve to hear what is being said of them. The instructions to kill themselves are not frightening since they may have thought of this for some time anyway.

The onset of voices in acute schizophrenia is often very frightening and the patient at times may attack the person he believes to be their source. Those with chronic schizophrenia on the other hand are often not troubled by the voices and may treat them as old friends, but a few patients complain bitterly about them. Those patients who are knowledgeable about their illness or who have insight into it may deny hallucinations, since they know this is an abnormal feature. Sometimes it is obvious that a patient is hallucinating if they stop talking and appear to be listening to something else or if they attempt to reply to the voices.

Body image distortions

Hyperschemazia, or the perceived magnification of body parts, can occur with a variety of organic and psychiatric conditions. When part of the body is painful it may feel larger than normal. When there is partial paralysis of a limb, the affected segment feels heavy and large, as in Brown–Sequard paralysis when the side with the extrapyramidal signs is hyperschematic, in peripheral vascular disease, in multiple sclerosis and following thrombosis of the posterior inferior cerebellar artery. In the latter two the hyperschemazia is unilateral. It may also occur in non-organic conditions such as hypochondriasis, depersonalisation and conversions disorder, and the distortion of image that is associated with feelings of fatness in anorexia nervosa is probably the best known.

The perception of body parts as absent or diminished is known as aschemazia or hyposchemazia respectively and is most likely to occur in parietal lobe lesions such as in thrombosis of the right middle cerebral artery, following transaction of the spinal cord or in health volunteers when underwater. Hyposchemazia must be distinguished from nihilistic delusions. Sims' (2003) comprehensive description of body image distortions cites Critchley (1950) as describing a patient with a parietal lobe infarct who had complex hyper- and hyposchemazia,

'It felt as if I was missing one side of my body (the left), but it also felt as if the dummy side was lined with a piece of iron so heavy that I could not move it … I even fancied my head to be narrow, but the left side from the centre felt heavy, as if filled with bricks'.

Koro or the belief that the penis is shrinking and will retract into the abdomen and cause death is found in South-East Asia and is thought to be due to a faulty understanding of anatomy. The diagnostic equivalent is probably anxiety disorder.

Paraschemazia or distortion of body image is described as a feeling that parts of the body are distorted or twisted or separated from the rest of the body and can occur in association with hallucinogenic use, with an epileptic aura and with migraine on rare occasions.

Hemisomatognosia is a unilateral lack of body image in which the person behaves as if one side of the body is missing and it occurs in migraine or during an epileptic aura. Anosognosia is 'denial of illness' and one study (Cutting, 1978) found that 58% of those with right hemisphere strokes denied their hemiplegia early after stroke and refused to admit to any weakness in their left arm. This belief typically remains despite manifest demonstration that it is paralysed. Some patients show bizarre attitudes to their paralysed limb, known as somatoparaphrenia (delusional beliefs about the body). They may have too many, they may be distorted, inanimate, severed or in other ways abnormal (Halligan *et al*, 1995). They may claim the limb belongs to a specified other person (Bisiach *et al*, 1991). Hemispatial neglect is the neglect of the hemispace on the contralateral side to the lesion when performing tasks, and a specific example, Gerstmann syndrome (lesion of dominant parietal lobe) consists of agraphia, acalculia, finger agnosia and right/left disorientation.

References

Bisiach, E., Rusconi, M. L. & Vallar, G. (1991) Remission of somatoparaphrenic delusion through vestibular stimulation. *Neuropsychologia*, **10**, 1029–1031.

Cooper, A. F. (1976) Deafness and psychiatric illness. *British Journal of Psychiatry*, **129**, 216–226.

Critchley, M. (1950) The body image in neurology. *Lancet*, **i**, 335–341.

Cutting, J. (1978) Study of anosognosia. *Journal of Neurology, Neurosurgery and Psychiatry*, **41**, 548–555.

Hamilton, M. (ed.) (1974) *Fish's Clinical Psychopathology. Signs and symptoms in Psychiatry*. Bristol: Wright.

Gonzalez-Pinto, A., van Os, J., Perez de Heredia, J. L., *et al* (2003) Age-dependence of Schniderian psychotic symptoms in bipolar patients. *Schizophrenia Research*, **61**, 157–162.

Halligan, P. W., Marshall, J. C. & Wade, D. T. (1995) Unilateral somatoparaphrenia after right hemisphere stroke: a case description. *Cortex*, **31**, 173–182.

Hamilton, M. (ed.) (1974) *Fish's Clinical Psychopathology. Signs and Symptoms in Psychiatry*. Bristol: John Wright and Sons Ltd.

Hare, E. H. (1973) A short note on pseudohallucinations. *British Journal of Psychiatry*, **122**, 289.

Jaspers, K. (1962) *General Psychopathology* (7th edn), (trans. J. Hoenig & M. W. Hamilton.) Manchester: Manchester University Press.

Leff, J. P. (1968) Perceptual phenomena and personality in sensory deprivation. *British Journal of Psychiatry*, **114**, 1499–1508.

Latcham, R. W., White, A. C. & Sims, A. C. P. (1978) Ganser syndrome: the aetiological argument. *Journal of Neurology, Neurosurgery and Psychiatry*, **41**, 851–854.

Manschreck, T. C., Maher, B. A., Winzig, L., *et al* (2000) Age disorientation in schizophrenia: an indicator of progressive and severe psychopathology, not institutional isolation. *Journal of Neuropsychiatry and Clinical Neurosciences*, **12**, 350–358.

Ohayon, M. M., Priest, R. G., Caulet, M., *et al* (1996) Hypnagogic and hypnopompic hallucinations: pathological phenomena? *British Journal of Psychiatry*, **169**, 459–467.

Pawar, A. V. & Spence, S. A. (2003) Defining thought broadcast. Semi-structured literature review. *British Journal of Psychiatry*, **183**, 287–291.

Sims, A. (2003) *Symptoms in the Mind. An introduction to Descriptive Psychopathology* (3rd edn). London: Saunders.

Tapp, A., Tandon, R., Scholten, R., *et al* (1993) Age disorientation in Kraepelinian schizophrenia: frequency and clinical correlates. *Psychopathology*, **26**, 225–228.

Ungvari, G. S. & Mullen, P. E. (1997) Reactive psychoses. In *Troublesome Disguises: Under-diagnosed Psychiatric Syndromes* (eds D. Bhugra & A. Munro). Oxford: Blackwell Science.

World Health Organization (1998) *Schedules for Clinical Assessment in Neuropsychiatry (SCAN)*. Geneva: WHO.

Disorders of thought and speech

Disorders of thought include disorders of intelligence, stream of thought and possession of thought, obsessions and compulsions and disorders of the content and form of thinking.

Disorders of intelligence

Intelligence is the ability to think and act rationally and logically. The measurement of intelligence is both complex and controversial (Ardila, 1999). In practice, intelligence is measured with tests of the ability of the individual to solve problems and to form concepts through the use of words, numbers, symbols, patterns and non-verbal material. The precise age at which intellectual growth appears to slow down depends on the type of test used, but it now appears that intelligence, as measured by intelligence tests, begins its slow decline in middle-age and proceeds significantly less rapidly than previously believed (McPherson, 1996).

The most common way of measuring intelligence is in terms of the distribution of scores in the population. The person who has an intelligence score on the 75 percentile has a score that is such that 75% of the appropriate population score less and 25% score more. Some intelligence tests used for children give a score in terms of the mental age, which is the score achieved by the average child of the corresponding chronological age. For historical reasons, most intelligence tests are designed to give a mean IQ of the population of 100 with a standard deviation of 15. Even if the distribution of scores is not normal, percentiles can be converted into standard units without difficulty and this is probably the best way of measuring intelligence.

Intelligence scores in a group of randomly chosen subjects of the same age tends to have a normal distribution, but this only applies over most of the range of scores. Towards the lower end of the range there is an increase in the incidence of low intelligence that is the result of brain damage caused by inherited disorders, birth trauma, infections and so on. There are, therefore, two groups of subjects with low intelligence or what is now termed 'learning disability' or 'intellectual disability'. The first group comprises individuals whose intelligence is at the lowest end of the normal range and is therefore a quantitative deviation from the normal. The other group of individuals with learning disability comprise individuals with specific learning disabilities. Many cases of learning disability are of unknown aetiology and thus, regardless of cause, learning disability tends to be categorised as borderline (IQ=70–90), mild (IQ=50–69), moderate (IQ=35–49), severe (IQ=20–34) and profound (IQ <20). More detailed clinical descriptions of these categories are provided in the ICD–10 *Classification of Mental and Behavioural Disorders* (World Health Organization, 1992).

Dementia is a loss of intelligence resulting from brain disease, characterised by disturbances of multiple cortical functions, including thinking, memory, comprehension and orientation, among others (World Health Organization, 1992). More detailed clinical and neuropathological accounts of dementias are provided by Lishman (1998). Individuals with schizophrenia tend to exhibit specific deficits in multiple cognitive domains (Sharma & Antonova, 2003) and these deficits have, in the past, been termed 'schizophrenic dementia'. These deficits do not, however, represent a true dementia and are best considered as part of the psychopathology of schizophrenia rather than as a form of dementia (McKenna *et al*, 1990). In particular, impairments of working and semantic memory seen in schizophrenia have been linked to dysfunction of the temporal cortex, frontal cortex and hippocampus (Kuperberg & Heckers, 2000); these impairments may have a significant impact on social functioning.

Disorders of thinking

The verb 'to think' is used rather loosely in English. Leaving aside such uses as 'to give an opinion' or 'to pay attention' there are three legitimate uses of the word 'think.' These are:

- undirected fantasy thinking (which, in the past, has also been termed autistic or dereistic thinking)
- imaginative thinking, which does not go beyond the rational and the possible
- rational thinking or conceptual thinking, which attempts to solve a problem.

It is obvious that the bounds between undirected fantasy thinking and imaginative thinking are not sharp, as it may be difficult to decide where fantasy ends and legitimate speculation begins. In the same way the boundary between imaginative thinking and rational thinking is not sharp.

Undirected fantasy or 'autistic' thinking

Undirected fantasy thinking is quite common, but certain individuals when faced with repeated disappointments or adverse life circumstances may engage in excessive undirected fantasy thinking. Bleuler (1911) believed that excessive 'autistic' thinking in schizophrenia was partly the result of formal thought disorder. Although the fantastic delusions of some individuals with chronic schizophrenia could be explained in this way, Bleuler's explanation is not helpful in describing or understanding all varieties of schizophrenia, and a more useful approach to thought form and content is presented below.

Classification of disorders of thinking

Any classification of disorders of thinking is bound to be arbitrary, at least to a certain extent. Thus it has been customary to divide thought disorders into disorders of content and disorders of form; or to put it into more familiar language, disorders of belief and disorders of reasoning. It is obvious that this division is somewhat artificial because belief and reasoning cannot be sharply separated. Apart from these two disorders, one can also consider disorders of the stream or progress of thought, which is also a somewhat arbitrary concept. Finally, there are disorders of the control of thinking, in which the subject is not in control of their thoughts, which may even be foreign to them. This might be considered as a disorder of volition or ego-consciousness. Realising that any division is bound to be arbitrary, it is suggested that for the sake of discussion we divide thought disorders into those of the stream of thought, the possession of thought, the content of thought and the form of thought.

Disorders of the stream of thought

Disorders of the stream of thought can be further divided into disorders of tempo and disorders of continuity.

Disorders of thought tempo

Flight of ideas

In flight of ideas thoughts follow each other rapidly; there is no general direction of thinking; and the connections between successive thoughts appear to be due to chance factors which, however, can usually be understood. The patient's speech is easily diverted to external stimuli and by internal superficial associations. The progress of thought can be compared to a game of dominoes in which one half of the first piece played determines one half of the next piece to be played. The absence of a determining tendency to thinking allows the associations of the train of thought to be determined by chance relationships, verbal associations of all kinds (such as assonance, alliteration and so on), clang associations, proverbs, maxims and clichés. The chance linkage of thoughts in flight of ideas is demonstrated by the fact that one could completely reverse the sequence of the record of a flight of ideas, and the progression of thought would be understood just as well.

An example of flight of ideas comes from a manic patient who was asked where she lived and she replied: 'Birmingham, Kingstanding; see the king he's standing, king, king, sing, sing, bird on the wing, wing, wing on the bird, bird, turd, turd.'

Flight of ideas is typical of mania. In hypomania so-called 'ordered flight of ideas' occurs in which, despite many irrelevances, the patient is able to return to the task in hand. In this condition clang and verbal associations are not so marked and the speed of emergence of thoughts is not as fast as in flight of ideas, so that this marginal variety of flight of ideas has been called 'prolixity.' Although these patients cannot keep accessory thoughts out of the main stream, they only lose the thread for a few moments and finally reach their goal. Unlike the tedious elaboration of details in circumstantiality, these patients have a lively embellishment of their thinking. In acute mania, flight of ideas can become so severe that incoherence occurs, because before one thought is formulated into words another forces its way forward.

Flight of ideas occasionally occurs in individuals with schizophrenia when they are excited and in individuals with organic states, including, for example, lesions of the hypothalamus, which are associated with a range of psychological effects, including features of mania and disturbances of personality (Lishman, 1998). What has been described so far is really flight of ideas with pressure of speech; it has been claimed that flight of ideas without pressure of speech occurs in some mixed affective states.

Inhibition or slowing of thinking

With inhibition or slowing of thinking, the train of thought is slowed down and the number of ideas and mental images that present themselves is decreased. This is experienced by the patient as difficulty in making decisions, lack of concentration and loss of clarity of thinking. There is also a diminution in active attention, so that events are poorly registered. This leads the patient to complain of loss of memory and to develop an overvalued or delusional idea that they are going out of their mind. The lack of concentration and the general fuzziness in thinking are often associated with a strange indescribable sensation 'in the head,' so that at times it is difficult to decide whether the patient is complaining about a physical or a psychiatric symptom. The apparent cognitive deficits in individuals with slowing of thinking in depression may lead to a mistaken diagnosis of dementia.

Slowing of thinking is seen in both depression and the rare condition of manic stupor. Many individuals with depression, however, may not have slowing of thinking but may experience difficulties with thinking owing to anxious preoccupations and increased distractibility due to anxiety.

Circumstantiality

Circumstantiality occurs when thinking proceeds slowly with many unnecessary and trivial details, but finally the point is reached. The goal of thinking is never completely lost and thinking proceeds towards it by an intricate and convoluted path. Historically, this disorder has been regarded as a feature of the constellation of personality traits occasionally associated with epilepsy (Kaplan & Saddock, 1996). Circumstantiality, however, can also occur in the context of learning disability and in individuals with obsessional personality traits.

Disorders of the continuity of thinking

Perseveration

Perseveration occurs when mental operations persist beyond the point at which they are relevant and thus prevent progress of thinking. Perseveration may be mainly verbal or ideational. Thus, a patient may be asked the name of the previous prime minister and reply 'John Major.' On being asked the name of the present prime minister he may reply 'John Major. No, I mean John Major.' This symptom is related to the severity of the task facing the patient, so that the more difficult the problem, the more likely it is that perseveration will occur. Perseveration is common in generalised and local organic disorders of the brain, and, when present, provides strong support for such a diagnosis.

In the early stages of perseveration, as in the above case, the patient may recognise their difficulty and try to overcome it. It is clear that this is not a problem of volition, which helps differentiate it from verbal stereotypy, which is a frequent spontaneous repetition of a word or phrase that is not in any way related to the current situation. In verbal stereotypy, the same word or phrase is used regardless of the situation, whereas in perseveration a word, phrase or idea persists beyond the point at which it is relevant.

Thought blocking

Thought blocking occurs when there is a sudden arrest of the train of thought, leaving a 'blank'. An entirely new thought may then begin. In patients who retain some insight, this may be a terrifying experience; this suggests that thought blocking differs from the more common experience of suddenly losing one's train of thought, which tends to occur when one is exhausted or very anxious. When thought blocking is clearly present it is highly suggestive of schizophrenia. However, patients who are exhausted and anxious may also lose the thread of the conversation and may appear to have thought blocking.

Obsessions, compulsions and disorders of the possession of thought

Normally one experiences one's thinking as being one's own, although this sense of personal possession is never in the foreground of one's consciousness. One also has the feeling that one is in control of one's thinking. In some psychiatric illnesses there is a loss of control or sense of possession of thinking.

Obsessions and compulsions

An obsession (also termed a rumination) is a thought that persists and dominates an individual's thinking despite the individual's awareness that the thought is either entirely without purpose or else has persisted and dominated their thinking beyond the point of relevance or usefulness. One of the most important features of obsessions is that their content is often of a nature as to cause the sufferer great anxiety and even guilt. The thoughts are particularly repugnant to the individual; thus the prudish person is tormented by sexual thoughts, the religious person by blasphemous thoughts, and the timid person by thoughts of torture, murder and general mayhem. It is of interest that the earlier writers emphasised the predominance of sexual obsessions, whereas nowadays it would appear that the most common forms of obsession tend to be concerned with fears of doing harm (for example, a mother with an obsession that she may harm her baby). This may reflect social change; the Victorians were particularly worried about sex, while modern man is more preoccupied with aggression and risk.

It is customary to distinguish between obsessions and compulsions. Compulsions are, in fact, merely obsessional motor acts. They may result from an obsessional impulse that leads directly to the action, or they may be mediated by an obsessional mental image or thought, as, for example, when the obsessional fear of contamination leads to compulsive washing.

The essential feature of the obsession is that it appears against the patient's will. It naturally follows that we can only call a mental event an obsession if it is normally under the control of the patient and can be resisted by the patient. Thus we have obsessional mental images, ideas, fears and impulses, but not obsessional hallucinations or moods.

Obsessional images are vivid images that occupy the patient's mind. At times they may be so vivid that they can be mistaken for pseudo-hallucinations. Thus one patient was obsessed by an image of his own gravestone that clearly had his name engraved on it. Obsessional ideas take the form of ruminations on all kinds of topics ranging from why the sky is blue to the possibility of committing fellatio with God. Sometimes obsessional thinking takes the form of contrast thinking in which the patient is compelled to think the opposite of what is said. This can be compulsive blasphemy, as, for example, in the case of the devout patient who was compelled to make blasphemous rhymes, so that when the priest said 'God Almighty' she was compelled to think 'Sod Allshitey'. Obsessional impulses may be impulses to touch, count or arrange objects, or impulses to commit antisocial acts. Apart from obsessions with suicide and homicide in depressed patients, it is very unusual for the obsessed patient to carry out an obsessive impulse. Obsessional fears or phobias consist of a groundless fear that the patient realises is dominating without a cause, and must be distinguished from the hysterical and learned phobias.

Obsessions occur in obsessional states, depression, schizophrenia, and occasionally in organic states; compulsive features appear to be particularly common in post-encephalitic parkinsonism (Lishman, 1998). In certain patients, there may be particular difficulties distinguishing obsessive–compulsive disorder from psychosis, as up to 14% of patients with obsessive–compulsive disorder may report psychotic phenomena such as delusions and hallucinations of thought disorder (Eisen & Rasmussen, 1993; Dowling *et al*, 1995). These psychotic or quasi-psychotic symptoms may have significant impact on the patient's ability to think clearly about their obsessions or compulsions (Kozak & Foa, 1994) and may, therefore, affect their ability to engage in cognitive or behavioural therapy.

Thought alienation

While the patient with obsession recognises that they are compelled to think about things against their will, they do not regard the obsessional thoughts as being foreign and outside their control. In thought alienation the patient has the experience that their thoughts are under the control of an outside agency or that others are participating in their thinking. In pure thought insertion the patient knows that thoughts are being inserted into their mind and they recognise them as being foreign and coming from without; this symptom, although commonly associated with schizophrenia, is not unique to schizophrenia, and a range of related phenomena have also been described (Mullins & Spence, 2003).

In thought deprivation, the patient finds that as they are thinking, their thoughts suddenly disappear and are withdrawn from thier mind by a foreign influence. It has been suggested that this is the subjective experience of thought blocking and 'omission'.

In thought broadcasting, the patient knows that as they are thinking, everyone else is thinking in unison with them. While this is the definition of thought broadcasting provided by Fish (Hamilton, 1974), there are also a number of other different definitions. For example, the term has been used to describe the belief that one's thoughts are quietly escaping from one's mind and that other people might be able to access them, and the experience of hearing one's thoughts spoken aloud and believing that, as a result, other people can hear them; these various definitions are reviewed by Pawar & Spence (2003). In clinical practice, it is useful to determine exactly what the patient believes with regard to their thoughts and to record it verbatim in the clinical notes. Experiences that resemble those described above can all be correctly described as thought broadcasting, but it is important to be aware that the term is used to describe a range of slightly different experiences.

In all these experiences of thought alienation the psychoanalytic interpretation is that the boundary between the ego and the surrounding world has broken down, so it is not altogether surprising that these symptoms were previously considered to be diagnostic of schizophrenia. Nowadays, thought alienation forms an important component of the diagnostic criteria for schizophrenia in the ICD−10 (World Health Organization, 1992).

These phenomena can be approached through the prism of ego-syntonicity/ego-dystonicity. An experience is described as ego-syntonic if it is consistent with the goals and needs of the ego and/or consistent with the individual's ideal self-image; the reverse is the case for ego-dystonicity. The division between ego-syntonic and ego-dystonic phenomena is not, however, absolute, and the clinical picture may be complicated by primary or secondary delusions, as well as changing mood states. In general, however, as an individual with psychosis develops insight into their symptoms, the experience of thought alienation may seem increasingly ego-dystonic and distressing to them.

Disorders of the content of thinking

It is customary to define a delusion as a false, unshakeable belief that is out of keeping with the patient's social and cultural background. The fact that a delusion is false makes it easy to recognise but this is not its essential quality. A very common delusion among married persons is that their spouses are unfaithful to them. In the nature of things, some of these spouses will indeed have been unfaithful; the delusion will therefore be true, but only by coincidence.

There is also a distinction between true delusions and delusion-like ideas. True delusions are the result of a primary delusional experience that cannot be deduced from any other morbid phenomenon, while the delusion-like idea is secondary and can be understandably derived from some other morbid psychological phenomenon – these are also described as secondary delusions (Sims, 1995).

Another important variety of false belief, which can occur in individuals both with and without mental illness, is the overvalued idea. This is a thought that, because of the associated feeling tone, takes precedence over all other ideas and maintains this precedence permanently or for a long period of time. Even though overvalued ideas tend to be less fixed than delusions and tend to have some degree of basis in reality, it may at times be difficult to distinguish between overvalued ideas and delusions (McKenna, 1984).

Primary delusions

It was previously held that primary delusional experiences were diagnostic of schizophrenia, although it is now recognised that similar experiences are described in other conditions, including certain organic states as well as psychotic illnesses.

The essence of the primary delusional experience (also termed apophany) is that a new meaning arises in connection with some other psychological event. Schneider (1959) suggested that these experiences can be reduced to three forms of primary delusional experience: delusional mood, delusional perception and the sudden delusional idea.

In the delusional mood the patient has the knowledge that there is something going on around him that concerns him, but he does not know what it is. Usually the meaning of the delusional mood becomes obvious when a sudden delusional idea or a delusional perception occurs. In the sudden delusional idea a delusion appears fully formed in the patient's mind. This is sometimes known as an autochthonous delusion. The form of this symptom is not in itself diagnostic of schizophrenia because sudden ideas or 'brain-waves' occur in individuals both with and without mental illness. In patients with depressive disorders or severe personality disorders sudden ideas of the nature of delusion-like ideas or overvalued ideas can occur. If a patient has a very grandiose or bizarre sudden idea, a diagnosis of schizophrenia should be actively considered.

The delusional perception is the attribution of a new meaning, usually in the sense of self-reference, to a normally perceived object. The new meaning cannot be understood as arising from the patient's affective state or previous attitudes. This last proviso is important because the delusional perception must not be confused with delusional misinterpretation. For example, a patient with delusions of persecution hears the stairs creak and knows that this is a detective spying on them. This is not a delusional perception, but a delusional misinterpretation. Schneider emphasised the importance of this symptom's 'two memberedness', as there is a link from the perceived object to the subject's perception of this object, and a second link to the new significance of this perception. Using this criterion, Schneider (1959) divided delusional memories into delusional perceptions and sudden delusional ideas. For example, if the patient says that they are of royal descent because they remember that the spoon they used as a child had a crown on it, this is really a delusional perception because there is the memory and also the delusional significance, i.e. the 'two memberedness'. On the other hand, if the patient says that they are of royal descent because when they were taken to a military parade as a small child the king saluted them, then this is a sudden delusional idea because the delusion is contained within the memory and there is no 'two memberedness'.

Primary delusional experiences tend to be reported in acute schizophrenia but are less common in chronic schizophrenia, where they may be buried under a mass of secondary delusions arising from primary delusional experiences, hallucinations, formal thought disorder and mood disorders.

Secondary delusions and systematisation

Secondary delusions can be understood as arising from some other morbid experience. Some authors have tried to explain all delusions as a result of some other morbid phenomenon. Psychoanalysts have stressed the role of projection in the formation of delusions, but as projection commonly occurs in individuals without psychosis, some other explanation is necessary to account for the excessive projection that occurs in delusions, particularly those of persecution. Sigmund Freud, for example, tried to explain delusions of persecution and grandeur as the result of latent homosexuality.

There is now considerable acceptance that delusions can be secondary to depressive moods and hallucinations, and that psychogenic or stress reactions can give rise to psychotic states with delusions; for example, acute polymorphic psychotic disorders in ICD−10 (World Health Organization, 1992) and brief psychotic disorder with stressor in the *Diagnostic and Statistical Manual of Mental Disorders* (DSM−IV; American Psychiatric Association, 1994). Personality can also play a role in the genesis of delusional states; abnormally suspicious personalities can react to difficulties with deepening ideas of persecution, or may slowly develop delusions of marital infidelity or bodily ill health. These latter disorders can be regarded as delusional disorders occurring on the background of personality disorder or abnormal personality traits.

Certain paranoid psychoses have been explained as 'understandable' developments of sensitive personalities (Jaspers, 1997). In this context, 'sensitive' means the patient is overly sensitive about some real or perceived psychological, social or physical failing that the patient felt held them back in some way. On this background, it is suggested that a full-blown paranoid psychosis may occur following a stressful event that refers to the perceived failing. This disorder, previously known as *sensitiver Beziehungswahn*, is now classified as a delusional disorder in the ICD–10 (World Health Organization, 1992).

In schizophrenia, once the primary delusional experiences have occurred they are commonly integrated into some sort of delusional system. This elaboration of delusions has been called 'delusional work.' It is still common among some practitioners to divide delusions into systematised and non-systematised. In the completely systematised delusions there is one basic delusion and the remainder of the system is logically built on this error. There may, however, be differing degrees of systematisation in different patients, and the level of systematisation may vary over time, with systematisation being generally more common in older patients or in patients whose delusions prove persistent.

The content of delusions

The content of delusions in schizophrenia is dependent, to a greater or lesser extent, on the social and cultural background of the patient. Common general themes include persecution, jealousy, love, grandiosity, ill health, guilt, nihilism and poverty. Specific delusional syndromes are outlined in Appendix I.

Delusions of persecution

Delusions of persecution may occur in the context of primary delusional experiences, auditory hallucinations, bodily hallucinations or experiences of passivity. Delusions of persecution can take many forms. In delusions of reference the patient knows that people are talking about him, slandering him or spying on him. It may be difficult to be certain if the patient has delusions of self-reference or if he has self-referential hallucinations. Ideas and delusions of reference are not confined to schizophrenia and can occur in depressive illness and other psychotic illnesses. Some patients with severe depression may believe that they are extremely wicked and that other people know this and are therefore quite justifiably spying on them. Delusions of guilt can be so marked that the patient believes that he is about to be put to death or imprisoned for life. This alleged persecution is generally believed to be fully justified by the patient. Occasionally, however, a patient may believe this alleged persecution is not justified and may attribute their depression to it. The supposed persecutors of the deluded patient may be people in the environment (such as members of the family, neighbours or former friends) or may be political or religious groups, of varying degrees of relevance to the patient.

Some patients believe that they or their loved ones are about to be killed, or are being tortured. In the latter case the delusions may be based on somatic hallucinations. The belief that the family is being harmed may be deduced from the content of the hallucinatory voices or the patient may claim that their relatives appear to be strange in some way and are obviously suffering from some interference. These symptoms may also be related to a perceptual or mood change in the patient. Some patients with delusions of persecution claim that they are being robbed or deprived of their just inheritance, while others claim they have special knowledge that their prosecutors wish to take from them.

Delusions of being poisoned or infected are not uncommon. Some patients who are morbidly jealous believe that their spouse is poisoning them. Often delusions of poisoning are explanatory delusions: the patient feels mentally and physically changed and the only way in which they can account for this is by assuming that their food or cigarettes have been poisoned. In other cases, delusions of poisoning are based on hallucinations of smell and taste.

Delusions of influence are a 'logical' result of experiences of passivity in the context of schizophrenia. These passivity feelings may be explained by the patient as the result of hypnotism, demonical possession, witchcraft, radio waves, atomic rays or television.

In day-to-day clinical practice it is common for the word 'paranoid' to be used as a substitute for the word 'persecutory,' but, strictly speaking, the correct meaning of the word paranoid is 'delusional.' Paranoia, which is the Greek for 'by the side of the mind,' was used in the late 19th century to designate functional mental illnesses in which delusions were the most prominent feature. The word paranoid was derived from this term and naturally had the meaning of 'like paranoia' or, in other words, delusional.

Delusions of infidelity

The commonly used term 'delusion of jealousy' is generally a misnomer as patients tend to have morbid jealousy with delusions of infidelity, rather than delusions of jealousy (Munro, 1999). Delusions of infidelity may occur in both organic and functional disorders. Often the patient has been suspicious, sensitive and mildly jealous before the onset of the illness. Delusions of marital infidelity are not uncommon in individuals with schizophrenia and have been reported in many different varieties of organic brain disorders, but are especially associated with alcohol dependency syndrome. Delusions of infidelity are also seen in the affective psychosis, where they may again represent a morbid exaggeration of a premorbid mildly jealous attitude.

Delusions of infidelity may develop gradually, as a suspicious or insecure person becomes more and more convinced of their spouse's infidelity and finally the idea reaches delusional intensity. The severity of the condition may also fluctuate over the course of time, and during episodes of marked disturbance, the spouse may be interrogated unceasingly and may be kept awake for hours at night. A jealous husband, for example, may interpret common phenomena as 'evidence' of infidelity; for example, he may insist that his wife has bags under her eyes as a result of frequent sexual intercourse with someone else, or may search his wife's underclothes for stains and claim that all stains are due to semen. This behaviour may progress to violence against the spouse and even to murder. Apart from delusions of infidelity, these patients tend not to show any other symptoms that would suggest schizophrenia.

Delusions of love

This condition has also been described as 'the fantasy lover syndrome' and 'erotomania'. The patient is convinced that some person is in love with them although the alleged lover may never have spoken to them (Kelly, 2005). They may pester the victim with letters and unwanted attention of all kinds (Kennedy et al, 2002). If there is no response to their letters, they may claim that their letters are being intercepted, that others are maligning them to their lover, and so on. Occasionally, isolated delusions of this kind are found in abnormal personality states. Sometimes, schizophrenia may begin with a circumscribed delusion of a fantasy lover and subsequently delusions may become more diffuse and hallucinations may develop.

Grandiose delusions

There is considerable variability in the extent of grandiosity associated with grandiose delusions in different patients. Some patients may believe they are God, the Queen of England, a famous rock star and so on. Others are less expansive and believe that they are skilled sportspersons or great inventors. The expansive delusions may be supported by auditory hallucinations, which tell the patient that they are important, or confabulations, when, for example, the patient gives a detailed account of their coronation or marriage to the king. Grandiose and expansive delusions may also be part of fantastic hallucinosis in which all forms of hallucination occur. In the past, delusions of grandeur were associated with 'general paralysis of the insane' (neurosyphilis) but are now most commonly associated with manic psychosis in the context of bipolar affective disorder. The patient may believe that they are an important person who is able to help others, or may report hearing the voice of God and the saints, confirming their elevated status.

Delusions of ill health

Delusions of ill health are a characteristic feature of depressive illnesses, but are also seen in other disorders, such as schizophrenia. Delusions of ill health may develop on a background of concerns about health; many people worry about their health and when they become depressed they naturally may develop delusions or overvalued ideas of ill health. This paradigm is similar to that advanced in the case of persecutory delusions, which may occur on a background of worry about one's relationships with others or suspiciousness about the intentions of other people. Such individuals, when depressed, may develop overvalued ideas or delusions of persecution.

Individuals with delusions of ill health in the context of depression may believe that they have a serious disease, such as cancer, tuberculosis, acquired immune-deficiency syndrome (AIDS), a brain tumour, and so on. Depressive delusions of ill health may involve the patient's spouse and children. Thus the depressed mother may believe that she has infected her children or that she is mad and her children have inherited incurable insanity. This may lead her to harm or even kill her children in the mistaken belief that she is putting them out of their misery. Many depressed puerperal women fear or believe that the newborn child has learning disabilities of some kind.

Delusions of ill health may take the form of primary or secondary delusions of incurable insanity. A significant number of individuals with depression may develop the belief that they are incurably insane. This may lead them to minimise their symptoms and refuse admission to psychiatric hospitals because they believe that they will spend the remainder of their life in an institution.

Hypochondriacal delusions in schizophrenia can be the result of a depressed mood, somatic hallucinations or a sense of subjective change. In the early stages, these delusions are usually the result of depression and may develop as mistaken explanations of psychological or physical symptoms. In individuals with chronic schizophrenia, they are usually the result of somatic hallucinations. Chronic hypochondriasis may also be linked to personality development. Insecure individuals may develop overvalued ideas of ill health that slowly increase in intensity and develop into delusions. These delusions may only become apparent following an operation or a complication of drug treatment.

Somewhat similar to these delusions are the delusional preoccupations with facial or bodily appearances, when the subject is convinced that their nose is too big, their face is twisted, or disfigured with acne, and so on. Sometimes these preoccupations with ill health or the appearance of the body have a somewhat obsessional quality, so that the patient cannot stop thinking about the supposed illness or deformity, although they realise it is ridiculous in times of quiet reflection. In other cases the belief is of delusional intensity and the patient is never able to admit that their belief is genuinely groundless. Contemporary classification systems tend to place some of these patients in the category of delusional disorders, which includes delusional dysmorphophobia (World Health Organization, 1992).

Delusions of guilt

In mild cases of depression the patient may be somewhat self-reproachful and self-critical. In severe depressive illness self-reproach may take the form of delusions of guilt, when the patient believes that they are a bad or evil person and have ruined their family. They may claim to have committed an unpardonable sin and insist that they will rot in hell for this. In very severe depression, the delusions may even appear to take on a grandiose character and the patient may assert that they are the most evil person in the world, the most terrible sinner who ever existed and that they will never die but will be punished for all eternity. These extravagant delusions of guilt are often associated with nihilistic ones. Furthermore, delusions of guilt may also give rise to delusions of persecution.

Nihilistic delusions

Nihilistic delusions or delusions of negation occur when the patient denies the existence of their body, their mind, their loved ones and the world around them. They may assert that they have no mind, no intelligence, or that their body or parts of their body do not exist; they may deny their existence as a person, or believe that they are dead, the world has stopped, or everyone else is dead. These delusions tend to occur in the context of severe, agitated depression and also in schizophrenia and states of delirium. Sometimes nihilistic delusions are associated with delusions of enormity, when the patient believes that they can produce a catastrophe by some action (e.g. they may refuse to urinate because they believe they will flood the world.

Delusions of poverty

The patient with delusions of poverty is convinced that they are impoverished and believe that destitution is facing them and their family. These delusions are typical of depression but appear to have become steadily less common over the past decades.

The reality of delusions

Not all individuals with delusions act on their delusional beliefs. Usually, when a delusional illness becomes chronic there is a discrepancy between the delusions and the patient's behaviour. For example, the grandiose patient who believes they are God may be happy to remain in a psychiatric hospital as a voluntary patient, or the persecuted patient who believes they are being poisoned may be happy to eat hospital food.

Depressive delusions of guilt and hypochondriasis may lead to action if the patient does not exhibit psychomotor retardation. Hypochondriacal delusions may lead to suicide or, if they involve the patient's family, homicide. Individuals with depression with severe delusions of guilt may try to give themselves up to the police. Delusions of infidelity are particularly dangerous and may be associated with violence or homicide (Munro, 1999). It is also possible that similar actions may be taken on the basis of delusion-like ideas or overvalued ideas, which may occur in individuals who do not have a major mental illness.

The pathology underlying delusions

Recent attempts to elucidate the precise forms of pathology underlying delusions have tended to focus on (a) developing models of the cognitive underpinnings of delusional beliefs and (b) using novel neuroimaging techniques to identify the brain areas or processes involved in developing and maintaining delusions.

From the cognitive perspective, for example, Huq et al (1988) have shown that individuals with delusions tend to make guesses based on less evidence than individuals with psychiatric illness who do not have delusions. In a related study, Garety et al (1991) found that individuals with delusions tended to change their minds more rapidly than individuals without delusions. Bentall (1990) has devised a useful heuristic model of the perceptual and cognitive processes involved in developing and maintaining beliefs and has expanded this model to address the development and maintenance of delusions (for an overview, see Bentall, 2003). Gilleen & David (2005) provide a valuable review of the cognitive neuropsychiatry of delusions, focusing on reasoning biases, attentional and attributional biases, and the relevance of emotion and theory of mind. In addition, they point to the role of functional neuroimaging techniques in exploring these areas in greater depth in the future.

From the neuroimaging perspective, various studies have suggested associations between types of delusions and different aspects of brain structure or function, including, for example, associations between abnormalities of cingulate gyrus activation and persecutory delusions (Blackwood et al, 2004), and between entorhinal cortex pathology and positive symptoms, especially delusions (Prasad et al, 2004). Blackwood et al (2000) suggest that anomalous connectivity or activity within defined brain regions may be related to the formation of delusions, while Szeszko et al (1999) point to a possible neurodevelopmental aspect to the aetiology of delusions. It is hoped that further work integrating both cognitive and neuroimaging approaches will shed greater light on the various pathologies that underlie delusions.

Disorders of the form of thinking

The term 'formal thought disorder' is a synonym for disorders of conceptual or abstract thinking that are most commonly seen in schizophrenia and organic brain disorders. In schizophrenia, disorders in the form of thinking may coexist with deficits in cognition (Sharma & Antonova, 2003), and these forms of thought disturbance may prove difficult to distinguish in certain cases. Bleuler (1911) regarded schizophrenia as a disorder of the associations between thoughts, characterised by the processes of condensation, displacement and misuse of symbols. In condensation, two ideas with something in common are blended into one false concept, while in displacement one idea is used for an associated idea. The faulty use of symbols involves using the concrete aspects of the symbol instead of the symbolic meaning ('concrete thinking').

Most other descriptions of formal thought disorder in schizophrenia describe the same phenomena in terms of different psychological concepts.

Cameron (1944), for example, used the term 'asyndesis' to describe the lack of adequate connections between successive thoughts. He pointed out that the patient with schizophrenia may demonstrate particular difficulty focusing on the issue at hand; may use imprecise expressions ('metonyms') instead of more exact ones; and may include excessive personal idiom and fantasy material in their speech. Cameron placed particular emphasis on 'over-inclusion', which is an inability to narrow down the operations of thinking and bring into action the organised attitudes and specific responses relevant to the task at hand. Goldstein (1944) emphasised the loss of abstract attitude in patients with schizophrenia, which leads to a 'concrete' style of thinking, despite the fact that the patient has not lost their vocabulary (unlike patients with organic brain disorders, for example).

Schneider (1930) claimed that five features of formal thought disorder could be identified: derailment, substitution, omission, fusion and drivelling. In derailment the thought slides on to a subsidiary thought, while in substitution a major thought is substituted by a subsidiary one. Omission consists of the senseless omission of a thought or part of it. In fusion, heterogeneous elements of thought are interwoven with each other, while in drivelling there is disordered intermixture of constituent parts of one complex thought. These disorders may be difficult to distinguish from each other in the clinical setting.

Schneider suggested there were three features of healthy thinking:

- constancy: this is characteristic of a completed thought that does not change in content unless and until it is superseded by another consciously-derived thought
- organisation: the contents of thought are related to each other in consciousness and do not blend with each other, but are separated in an organised way
- continuity: there is a continuity of the sense continuum, so that even the most heterogenous subsidiary thoughts, sudden ideas or observations that emerge are arranged in order in the whole content of consciousness.

Schneider claimed that individuals with schizophrenia complained of three different disorders of thinking that correspond to these three features of normal or non-disordered thinking. These were: a peculiar transitoriness of thinking, the lack of normal organisation of thought, and desultory thinking. There were three corresponding varieties of objective thought disorder, as follows:

Transitory thinking

Transitory thinking is characterised by derailments, substitutions and omissions. Omission is distinguished from desultory thinking because in desultoriness the continuity is loosened but in omission the intention itself is interrupted and there is a gap. The grammatical and syntactical structures are both disturbed in transitory thinking.

Drivelling thinking

With drivelling thinking, the patient has a preliminary outline of a complicated thought with all its necessary particulars, but loses preliminary organisation of the thought, so that all the constituent parts get muddled together. The patient with drivelling have a critical attitude towards their thoughts, but these are not organised and the inner material relationships between them become obscured and change in significance.

Desultory thinking

In desultory thinking speech is grammatically correct but sudden ideas force their way in from time to time. Each one of these ideas is a simple thought that, if used at the right time would be quite appropriate.

Speech disorders

Disorders of speech are seen in a broad range of psychiatric and neurological disorders. They include stammering and stuttering, mutism, talking past the point, neologisms, schizophasia and aphasia.

Stammering and stuttering

In stammering the normal flow of speech is interrupted by pauses or by the repetition of fragments of the word. Grimacing and tic-like movements of the body are often associated with stammer. Stuttering usually begins at about the age of 4 years and is more common in boys than girls. Often it improves with time (World Health Organization, 1992) and may only become noticeable when the person is anxious for any reason. Sometimes it persists into adult life when it may be a significant social disability. Occasionally stammering occurs during a severe adolescent crisis or at the onset of acute schizophrenia. This is probably the result of severe anxiety bringing to light a childhood stammer that has been successfully overcome.

Mutism

Mutism is the complete loss of speech and may occur in children with a range of emotional or psychiatric disorders and in adults with hysteria, depression, schizophrenia or organic brain disorders. Elective mutism may occur in children who refuse to speak to certain people; for example, the child may be mute at school but speak at home. In certain families, refusal to speak may become a recognised technique for dealing with family quarrels. Occasionally, there are families in which some members have not spoken for years though they live under the same roof.

Hysterical mutism is relatively rare and the most common hysterical disorder of speech is aphonia. Severe depression with psychomotor retardation may be associated with mutism, but more often there is poverty of speech and the patient replies to questions in a slow and drawn-out fashion. Mutism is almost always present in catatonic stupor, but it may also occur in non-stuperose catatonic individuals as a mannerism. Thus in 1935 a catatonic patient said 'My words are too valuable to be given away' and thereafter she never spoke a word. When she was seen 20 years later she was still mute, but she would make her wants known by gesture and at times she would write the answers to questions when given a pencil and paper.

Although the use of words is very restricted in severe motor aphasia, complete mutism does not occur, because the patient may use one or more verbal stereotypies and may use expletives under emotional stress. In pure word-dumbness the patient is mute but can and will read and write. In akinetic mutism, which is associated with lesions of the upper midbrain or posterior diencephalon (Lishman, 1998), there is mutism and the patient appears to be aware of the environment, despite a lowering of the level of consciousness and anterograde amnesia.

Talking past the point (Vorbeireden)

In this disorder the content of the patient's replies to questions shows that they understand what has been asked but have responded by talking about an associated topic. For example, if asked 'What is the colour of grass?', the patient may reply 'White', and if then asked 'What is the colour of snow?', they may reply 'Green'. One patient when asked the year when the First World War began gave their year of birth and when asked for the year of their birth replied '1914'. Talking past the point occurs in hysterical pseudodementia (now classified as a dissociative or conversion disorder) when psychiatric symptoms are 'unconsciously' being presented for some advantage. 'Approximate answers' may be a feature of Ganser's syndrome, which is another dissociative or conversion disorder that tends to occur in circumstances that indicate a psychogenic aetiology (World Health Organization, 1992).

Talking past the point is also found in acute schizophrenia, especially among adolescents. The adolescent patient may find the phenomenon amusing and assume a facetious attitude towards it, consistent with the hebephrenic subtype of schizophrenia. This is also known as 'pseudodementia.' Individuals in catatonic states may also talk past the point, particularly when asked personal questions that they find painful, such as the length of their stay in hospital.

Neologisms

Neologisms may be new words that are constructed by the patient or ordinary words that are used in a new way. The term 'neologism' is usually applied to new word formations produced by individuals with schizophrenia. Some patients with aphasia, particularly those with motor aphasia, use the wrong word, invent new words, or distort the phonetic structure of words. This is usually known as paraphasia, though superficially the words resemble neologisms. When an individual with schizophrenia produces a new word it may be completely new and its derivation cannot be understood; it may be a distortion of another word; or it may be a word that has been incorrectly constructed by the faulty use of the accepted rules of word formation.

Neologisms in individuals with catatonia may be mannerisms or stereotypies. The patient may distort the pronunciation of some words in the same way as they distort some movements of their body. Some patients use a stock word instead of the correct one. For example, a patient may use the word 'car' and call an airplane an 'air car' and a boat a 'sea car'. In other cases neologisms appear to be a result of a severe positive formal thought disorder, so that words are fused together in the same way as concepts are blended with one another. Alternatively, the neologism may be the obvious result of a derailment; for example, a patient used the word 'relativity' instead of the word 'relationship.' In other cases the neologism seems to be an attempt to find a word for an experience that is completely outside the realms of normal. This can be called a technical neologism because the patient is making up a technical term for a private experience that cannot be expressed in ordinary words. In other patients hallucinatory voices seem to play a great part in the formation of neologisms. The 'voices' may use neologisms and this may lead the patient to use them as well. Sometimes the patient feels forced to use new words in order to placate the 'voices' or to protect themself from them.

Malapropisms, which are conspicuously misused words, may be mistaken for neologisms in some individuals, but are, themselves, of no particular known psychiatric significance.

Speech confusions and schizophasia

Some individuals with schizophrenia produce speech that is profoundly confused but are, none the less, able to carry out responsible work that does not involve the use of words. Schizophasia has a superficial resemblance to aphasia, where the disorder of speech is much greater than the deficit in intelligence. Despite the apparent discrepancy between thought and speech, schizophasia is generally regarded as a form of thought disorder. Schizophasia is also known as 'speech confusion' and 'word salad'.

Speech disorders in schizophrenia have received considerable research attention in recent years, and there is now evidence that the speech of individuals with schizophrenia not only displays many of the classical phenomena described above (for example, schizophasia), but is also, overall, syntactically less complex than that of controls (Thomas *et al*, 1996). While this poor linguistic performance appears to be more related to the illness process rather than the effects of institutionalisation (Thomas *et al*, 1990), this is certainly an area that merits further study.

Aphasia

Aphasia or dysphasia is a disorder of speech resulting from interference with the functioning of certain areas of the brain. This brief discussion of aphasia has been included in order that the disorders of speech associated with major psychiatric disorders (such as schizophrenia) can be compared to those that, like the aphasias, are more likely to have an organic origin (such as brain tumours and lesions of various descriptions). For a more detailed examination of the organic and clinical aspects of aphasia, the reader is referred to Lishman (1998). In clinical practice, aphasias tend to be classified into three groups, as follows.

Receptive aphasias

Three types of aphasia can be regarded as receptive: pure word deafness, agnostic alexia and visual asymbolia. In pure word deafness the patient hears words but cannot understand them; this is generally attributable to a lesion in the dominant temporal lobe. In agnosic alexia the patient can see but cannot read words; this is generally attributable to lesions of the left visual cortex and the corpus callosum.

In visual asymbolia or cortical visual aphasia there is disorganisation of visual word schemas so that words cannot be recognised and motor word schemas cannot be activated; this is generally attributable to lesions involving the angular and supramarginal gyri. The patient with visual asymbolia finds it difficult to read and write. As the lesion may be extensive and affect neighbouring structures, this variety of aphasia is often associated with other neurological disorders such as inability to use mathematical symbols (acalculia), spatial disorientation, visual agnosia, nominal aphasia and right homonymous hemianopia. Patients with visual asymbolia are often able to understand words or sentences that they cannot read aloud or that they read aloud incorrectly. Unlike patients with agnostic alexia they can copy writing to some extent but have difficulty in writing spontaneously.

The agnosias are related to the receptive aphasias. In these disorders the patient experiences sensation in a given modality but they cannot recognise objects. Thus, in visual agnosia the patient can see but cannot recognise what they see, although they can recognise objects if they feel them. Patients with agnosia can neither describe nor use the object, so that there is both an aphasia and an apraxia. A detailed discussion of agnosias is not possible in the present text (see Lishman, 1998), but it should be remembered that these conditions may be mistakenly regarded as a dissociative or conversion disorder if they occur in isolation.

Intermediate aphasias

In nominal (amnesic) aphasia the patient cannot name objects, although they have plenty of words at their disposal. Usually they find it difficult to carry out verbal and written commands and they cannot write spontaneously, although as a rule they can copy written material. Difficulty in finding the correct word can occur in other varieties of aphasia, but in nominal aphasia it is the outstanding disorder. Nominal aphasia may be found with either diffuse brain damage or with focal lesions involving, for example, the dominant temporoparietal region.

In central (conduction) aphasia the patient experiences substantial disturbances in language function with impairments of speech and writing. Speech is faulty in grammar and syntax and there is paraphasia. Both the receptive and expressive aspects of speech may be affected. This disorder is also known as 'syntactical aphasia' and may result from a number of different lesions (Lishman, 1998).

Expressive aphasias

The main type of expressive aphasia is cortical motor aphasia, which is also known as Broca's aphasia, verbal aphasia or expressive aphasia. It is usually caused by lesions of Broca's area in the posterior two-thirds of the third frontal convolution, but it can also result from lesions affecting the association fibres that run forward from the speech centre in the first temporal convolution. In this type of aphasia the patient has difficulty putting their thoughts into words and in severe cases speech may be restricted to expletives and a few words. The patient may use only one word, a paraphasic word, a phrase, or either 'yes' or 'no' or both these words. Frequently if a phrase is used it was present in the patient's mind when the lesion occurred. Often these 'recurring utterances' or verbal stereotypies are produced with different intonations to produce different meanings.

When the disorder is less severe the patient understands what is said to them and knows what they want to say but cannot find the right words. Words are often mispronounced and those with several syllables tend to be abbreviated. As a rule the patient realises that they are making mistakes and tries to correct them. Although words are often omitted, the organisation of sentences is not as severely affected as the use of words. The omission of articles and short words gives rise to a 'telegram style' of speech. Serial responses are often not affected, so that the patient may be able to count, recite the alphabet and give the days of the week. The expressive quality of speech is disordered, so that the intonation and stress are unusual and speech sounds stilted and odd. Usually the patient can swear and say words under emotional stress.

In pure word-dumbness the patient is unable to speak spontaneously, to repeat words and to read aloud, but they can write spontaneously, copy and write to dictation. This disorder probably results from a lesion beneath the region of the insula (Lishman, 1998).

References

American Psychiatric Association (1994) *Diagnostic and Statistical Manual of Mental Disorders* (4th edn) (DSM–IV). Washington, DC: APA.

Ardila, A. (1999) A neuropsychological approach to intelligence. *Neuropsychology Review,* **9**, 117−136

Bentall, R. P. (ed.) (1990) *Reconstructing Schizophrenia.* London: Routledge.

Bentall, R. P. (2003) *Madness Explained: Psychosis and Human Nature.* London: Allen Lane.

Blackwood, N. J., Howard, R. J., Ffytche, D. H., *et al* (2000) Imaging attentional and attributional bias: an fMRI approach to the paranoid delusion. *Psychological Medicine,* **30**, 873−883.

Blackwood, N. J., Bentall, R. P., Ffytche, D. H., *et al* (2004) Persecutory delusions and the determination of self-relevance: an fMRI investigation. *Psychological Medicine,* **34**, 591−596.

Bleuler, E. (1911) *Dementia Praecox or the Group of Schizophrenias.* Reprinted 1950 (trans. & ed. J. Zinkin). New York: International University Press.

Cameron, N. (1944) Experimental analysis of schizophrenic thinking. In *Language and Thought in Schizophrenia* (ed. J. Kasanin). Berkeley, CA: University of California Press.

Dowling, F. G., Pato, M. T., & Pato, C. N. (1995) Comorbidity of obsessive−compulsive and psychotic symptoms: a review. *Harvard Review of Psychiatry,* **3**, 75−83.

Eisen, J. L. & Rasmussen, S. A. (1993) Obsessive−compulsive disorder with psychotic features. *Journal of Clinical Psychiatry,* **54**, 373−379.

Garety, P. A, Hemsley, D. R., & Wessely, S. (1991) Reasoning in deluded schizophrenia and paranoid patients. *Journal of Nervous and Mental Disease,* **179**, 194−201.

Gilleen, J. & David, A. S. (2005) The cognitive neuropsychiatry of delusions: from psychopathology to neuropsychology and back again. *Psychological Medicine,* **35**, 5−12.

Goldstein, K. (1944) Methodological approach to the study of schizophrenic thought disorder. In *Language and Thought in Schizophrenia* (ed. J. Kasanin). Berkeley, CA: University of California Press.

Hamilton, M. (1974) *Fish's Clinical Psychopathology.* Bristol: Wright.

Huq, S. F., Garety, P. A., & Hemsley, D. R. (1988) Probabilistic judgements in deluded and nondeluded subjects. *Quarterly Journal of Experimental Psychology,* **40A**: 801−812.

Jaspers, K. (1997) *General Psychopathology* (trans. J. Hoenig & M. W. Hamilton). Baltimore: Johns Hopkins University Press.

Kaplan, H. I. & Saddock, B. J. (1996) *Concise Textbook of Clinical Psychiatry* (7th edn). Baltimore,: Williams & Wilkins.

Kelly, B. D. (2005) Erotomania − epidemiology and management. *CNS Drugs,* **19**, 657−669.

Kennedy, N., McDonagh, M., Kelly, B., *et al* (2002) Erotomania revisited: clinical course and treatment. *Comprehensive Psychiatry,* **43**, 1−6.

Kozak, M. J. & Foa, E. B. (1994) Obsessions, overvalued ideas, and delusions in obsessive-compulsive disorder. *Behaviour Research and Therapy,* **32**, 343−353.

Kuperberg, G. & Heckers, S. (2000) Schizophrenia and cognitive function. *Current Opinion in Neurobiology,* **10**, 205−210.

Lishman, W. A. (1998) *Organic Psychiatry: The Psychological Consequences of Cerebral Disorder* (3rd edn). Oxford: Blackwell Science.

McKenna, P. J. (1984) Disorders with overvalued ideas. *British Journal of Psychiatry,* **145**, 579−585.

McKenna, P. J., Tamlyn, D., Lund, C. E., *et al* (1990) Amnesic syndrome in schizophrenia. *Psychological Medicine,* **20**, 967−972.

McPherson, F. M. (1996) Psychology in relation to psychiatry. In *Companion to Psychiatric Studies* (5th edn) (eds, R. E. Kendell & A. K. Zealley). Edinburgh: Churchill Livingstone.

Mullins, S. & Spence, S. A. (2003) Re-examining thought insertion: semi-structured literature review and conceptual analysis. *British Journal of Psychiatry,* **182**, 293−298.

Munro, A. (1999) *Delusional Disorder: Paranoia and Related Illnesses.* Cambridge: Cambridge University Press.

Pawar, A. V. & Spence, S. A. (2003) Defining thought broadcast: semi-structured literature review. *British Journal of Psychiatry,* **183**, 287−291.

Prasad, K. M., Patel, A. R., Muddasani, S., *et al* (2004) The entorhinal cortex in first-episode psychotic disorders: a structural magnetic resonance imaging study. *American Journal of Psychiatry*, **161**, 1612–1619.

Schneider, C. (1930) [*Psychologie der Schizopheren*] (Psychology of Schizophrenics). Leipzig: Thieme.

Schneider, K. (1959) *Clinical Psychopathology* (trans. M. Hamilton) New York: Grune & Stratton.

Sharma, T. & Antonova, L. (2003) Cognitive function in schizophrenia. Deficits, functional consequences, and future treatment. *Psychiatric Clinics of North America*, **26**, 25–40.

Sims, A. (1995) *Symptoms in the Mind: An Introduction to Descriptive Psychopathology* (2nd edn). London: Saunders.

Szeszko, P. R., Bilder, R. M., Lencz, T., *et al* (1999) Investigation of frontal lobe subregions in first-episode schizophrenia. *Psychiatry Research*, **90**, 1–15.

Thomas, P., King, K., Fraser, W. I., *et al* (1990) Linguistic performance in schizophrenia: a comparison of acute and chronic patients. *British Journal of Psychiatry*, **156**, 204–210.

Thomas, P., Kearney, G., Napier, E., *et al* (1996) Speech and language in first onset psychosis differences between people with schizophrenia, mania, and controls. *British Journal of Psychiatry*, **168**, 337–343.

World Health Organization (1992) *The ICD–10 Classification of Mental and Behavioural Disorders: Clinical descriptions and diagnostic guidelines* (10th edn). Geneva: WHO.

CHAPTER 4

Disorders of memory

Memory is of three types: sensory, short-term and long-term. It can be compared to a sieve with holes of varying size to assist in identifying material that is relevant from that which is irrelevant. The first, known as sensory memory, is registered for each of the senses and its purpose is to facilitate the rapid processing of incoming stimuli so that comparisons can be made with material already stored in short- and long-term memory. Since there are numerous stimuli bombarding the individual, selective attention allows for the sifting of relevant material from sensory memory for further processing and storage in short-term memory. As a consequence, most sensory memory fades within a few seconds. Short-term memory, also called working memory, allows for the storage of memories for much longer than the few seconds available to sensory memory. Short-term memory aids the constant updating of one's surroundings. For example, if you saw a person walking a dog and a few seconds later heard a dog bark you would not be surprised since you would identify the likely source of the sound from sensory (visual) memory that had been processed and encoded in short-term (working) memory.

When memories have been rehearsed in short-term memory they are encoded into long-term memory. Encoding is the process of placing information into what is believed to be a limitless memory reservoir, which can occur for specific stimuli as well as for the general memory. For example, passing a large two-storey house painted yellow with a tennis court and two sports cars in front might be recalled exactly (visual encoding) or recalled in more general terms as the large home of a wealthy owner (semantic encoding).

The storage of material in long-term memory allows for recall of events from the past and for the utilisation of information learned through the education system. It is resilient to attack, unlike short-term memory, which is sensitive to disorders of brain tissue such as Alzheimer's disease.

Autobiographical memory refers to the memories for events and issues that relate to oneself. These may be for specific facts, for example whether you are you married, and specific experiences, for example your wedding day.

It is characterised by a general recall of the event, an interpretation of the event and a recall of a few specific details. Flashbulb memories are a specific type of autobiographical memory in which the person becomes aware of an emotionally arousing event, for example the 9/11 terrorist bombings. Even though they are recalled with seeming accuracy due to rehearsal, their accuracy cannot be assumed.

Autobiographical memories in general are not necessarily like video-playbacks since they may represent the personal meaning and interpretation that the event had for the person at the expense of accuracy. Autobiographical memories are associated with the active experience of remembering.

Most memory tests measure recall of prior events either from the person's life or from tests that were administered earlier. Common clinical examples of this are 5-minute recalls, asking the patient what they had for breakfast or inquiring about details of their past life. In responding to such inquiries the person is conscious that they are remembering. This is known as explicit or declarative or relational memory and is of two types: episodic memory or memory for specific events, for example going to the shops this morning, and semantic memory or memory for abstract facts such as 'What the capital of Chad?' Autobiographical memory is one type of episodic memory.

However, the performance of tasks such as typing, swimming or cutting a loaf of bread are also expressions of prior learning but there is no active awareness that memory is being searched in undertaking the particular skill. This type of memory is known as implicit or procedural or skills memory.

Studies of people with injury to the hippocampus suggest that declarative and procedural memory use different parts of the brain and can function independently. The hippocampus is believed to be the site where explicit (procedural) memory is stored, while implicit (declarative) memory is thought to reside in the limbic system, the amygdala and the cerebellum. For example, when a person with damage to the hippocampus is repeatedly retrained in a task, although there may be a recollection of this, there is no concomitant improvement in skills; thus they have functioning declarative memory but damaged procedural memory.

The process of remembering has four parts: registration, retention, retrieval and recall. For the purposes of discussion we can divide memory impairments into amnesias (loss of memory) and paramnesias (distortions of memory).

The amnesias

Amnesia is defined as partial or total inability to recall past experiences and events and its origin may be organic or psychogenic.

Failure to recall may also occur due to normal memory decay, so that if an item is not rehearsed the memory fades and thereafter cannot be retrieved. Many people incorrectly assume that memory is like a cine-camera, replaying material exactly as recorded and therefore representing a perfect match to events from the past. This carries huge implications, especially when giving evidence about past events in the courts and is one of the reasons for a statute of limitations applying to some civil and criminal cases. A further cause of normal memory failure is interference from related material. In proactive interference old memories interfere with new learning and hence with recall, while in retroactive interference new memories interfere with the retrieval of old material. Proactive interference explains why learning Spanish this year will make it difficult to learn German next year, while retroactive interference explains why learning Spanish this year makes it difficult to recall the German learned least year.

Psychogenic amnesias

Dissociative or hysterical amnesia is the sudden amnesia that occurs during periods of extreme trauma and can last for hours or even days. The amnesia will be for personal identity such as name, address and history as well as for personal events, while at the same time the ability to perform complex behaviours is maintained. There is a discrepancy between the marked memory impairment and the preservation of personality and social skills, so that the person behaves appropriately to their background and education. Dissociation may be associated with a fugue or wandering state in which the subject travels to another town or country and is often found wandering and lost. There are descriptions of dissociative amnesia occurring in those charged with serious offences, although in these circumstances the distinction from malingering is difficult to make. Dissociative amnesia is believed to be more common in those with a prior history of head injury.

The more limited amnesia for specific traumatic events is known as katathymic amnesia or motivated forgetting, though the terms are often used interchangeably with dissociative amnesia. Katathymic amnesia is the inability to recall specific painful memories, and is believed to occur due to the defence mechanism of repression (described in 1895 by Freud, Breuer and colleagues; Freud *et al*, 1895) (for definition of repression see Appendix II). However, it is unclear whether the repression is driven by a conscious motivation to forget, i.e. suppression, or whether it is unconscious, i.e. primary repression. Katathymic amnesia is more persistent and circumscribed than dissociation in that there is no loss of personal identity. In this state the traumatic incident is not available to recall unless some trigger or psychotherapeutic intervention makes the memory available to consciousness, a view that is itself controversial. This amnesia is believed to last for many years and is said to underpin recovered memory syndrome (Bass & Davis, 1988), although this view is challenged by those who dispute its existence (Loftus, 1993) preferring to call it false memory syndrome (see paramnesia below). A detailed review of traumatic amnesia is provided by Brewin & Andrews (1998).

Organic amnesias

Acute brain disease

In these conditions memory is poor owing to disorders of perception and attention. Hence there is a failure to encode material in long-term memory. In acute head injury there is an amnesia, known as retrograde amnesia, that embraces the events just before the injury. This period is usually no longer than a few minutes but occasionally may be longer, especially in subacute conditions. Anterograde amnesia is amnesia for events occurring after the injury. These occur most commonly following accidents and are indicative of failure to encode events into long-term memory. Blackouts are circumscribed periods of anterograde amnesia experienced particularly by those who are alcohol dependent during and following bouts of drinking. They indicate reversible brain damage and vary in length but can span many hours. They also occur in acute confusional states (delirium) due to infections or epilepsy.

Subacute coarse brain disease

The characteristic memory disorder is the amnestic state in which the patient is unable to register new memories. The memory disorder is characterised by the inability to learn new information (anterograde amnesia), and the inability to recall previously learned material (retrograde amnesia). However, memories from the remote past remain intact, as does recall of over learned material from the past and immediate recall. As improvement occurs, the amnestic period may shrink and recovery may sometimes be total. This diagnosis is not made when there are other signs of cognitive impairment as in dementia or when consciousness is clouded as in delirium. Korsakoff's syndrome is the amnestic syndrome caused by thiamine deficiency, but other causes include cerebrovascular disease, multiple sclerosis, transient global amnesia, head injury and electroconvulsive treatment (ECT).

Chronic coarse brain disease

Patients with amnesia or those with Korsakoff's syndrome usually have a loss of memory extending back into the recent past for a year or so. Patients with a progressive chronic brain disease have an amnesia extending over many years, though the memory for recent events is lost before that for remote events. This was pointed out by Ribot and is known as Ribot's law of memory regression.

Other amnesias

Anxiety amnesia occurs when there is anxious preoccupation or poor concentration in disorders such as depressive illness or generalised anxiety. Initially it may wrongly suggest dissociative amnesia. More severe forms of amnesia in depressive disorders resemble dementia and are known as depressive pseudodementia. Amnesias in anxiety and depressive disorders are generally caused by impaired concentration and resolve once the underlying disorder is treated.

Distortions of memory or paramnesia

This is the falsification of memory by distortion and can be conveniently divided into distortions of recall and distortions of recognition. This can occur in normal subjects due to the process of normal forgetting or due to proactive and retroactive interference from newly acquired material. It can occur in those with emotional problems as well as in organic states.

Distortions of recall

Retrospective falsification

Retrospective falsification refers to the unintentional distortion of memory that occurs when it is filtered through a person's current emotional, experiential and cognitive state. It is often found in those with depressive illness who describe all past experiences in negative terms due to the impact of their current mood. So a depressed person will highlight their failures while ignoring and/or forgetting about their successes. This may give the impression that the person has always been incompetent and unstable. Indeed any psychiatric illness can lead to retrospective falsification. Even following recovery the falsification may continue, as for example when a person following discharge from hospital exaggerates the restrictions that were placed upon them, while forgetting the necessity of such measures. This is invariably related to the insight of the patient as well as to suggestibility. Those with hysterical personality, in whom suggestibility is high, can therefore produce a complete set of distorted memories of the past.

False memory

False memory is the recollection of an event (or events) that did not occur but which the individual subsequently strongly believes did take place (Brandon *et al*, 1998). The syndrome refers not to distortion of true memories, as in normal forgetting, but to the actual construction of memories around events that never took place. Although this definition was developed specifically in the context of childhood abuse recalled by adults, it can also be applied in rare situations, such as false confessions to serious crimes (Gudjonsson *et al*, 1999). The origin of this latter false memory is termed memory distrust syndrome and emanates from the person's own fundamental distrust of their memory, termed 'source amnesia'. This source amnesia (Johnson *et al*, 1993) arises because of difficulty remembering the source from which the information was acquired, whether from one's own recall or from some external source as recounted by others. In view of the fallibility of memory this phenomenon should hardly be surprising. For example, healthy people have trouble remembering the source of much information, including when, where, from whom or in what modality (spoken or written). This difficulty worsens with increasing age and is an even greater problem in the presence of organic brain disease. Those who are suggestible are also at greater risk of false memory. In these instances it is important to identify an actual memory since it is possible to have false belief without any memory (Gudjonsson, 1997), as for example in a person who says they were in hospital following a cerebrovascular accident (CVA) when in fact they had no recollection of this and had been told by their family that it had happened.

Screen memory

A screen memory is a recollection that is partially true and partially false; it is thought that the individual only recalls part of the true memory because the entirety of the true memory is too painful to recall. For example, an individual may recall that childhood sexual abuse was perpetrated by a neighbour because it is too painful to recall that the abuse was, in fact, perpetrated by their own brother. In any given case, it is difficult to dissect out precisely which elements of such memories are objectively true; this may be important in both the therapeutic and legal settings. The relationships between screen memories, psychological symptoms and other psychic phenomena (such as dreams) may be difficult to establish, but untangling these relationships may be seen as an opportunity for psychological or psychoanalytic exploration in certain cases (Good, 1998; Battin & Mahon, 2003).

Confabulation

Confabulation is the falsification of memory occurring in clear consciousness in association with organic pathology. It manifests itself as the filling-in of gaps in memory by imagined or untrue experiences that have no basis in fact. Some of the statements may be contradictory yet no attempt is made to correct them. The confabulation diminishes as the impairment worsens. Two broad patterns emerge (Bonhoeffer, 1901), the embarrassed type in which the patient tries to fill in gaps in memory as a result of an awareness of a deficit and the fantastic type in which the lacunae are filled in by details exceeding the need of the memory impairment such as descriptions of wild adventures. Overall the embarrassed type is much more common and it may represent real memories displaced in time. Some schizophrenics confabulate and provide detailed descriptions of fantastic events that have never happened. Some suggest that confabulation is a misnomer since these memories are fixed and unchanging. The term pictorial thinking is used instead by some, while others call them memory hallucinations, a term rejected by Fish as 'not very suitable'. They may best be termed retrospective delusions (see below). Lethologia, the temporary inability to remember names or proper nouns, is common and generally not indicative of any pathology.

Pseudologia fantastica

Pseudologia fantastica or fluent plausible lying (pathological lying) is the term used, by convention, to describe the confabulation that occurs in those without organic brain pathology such as personality disorder of antisocial or hysterical type. Typically the subject describes various major events and traumas or makes grandiose claims and these often present at a time of personal crisis, such as facing legal proceedings. Although it seems that the person with pseudologia believes their own stories and there is a blurring of the boundary between fantasy and reality, when confronted with incontrovertible evidence these individuals will admit their lying. Minor varieties of this occur in those who falsify or exaggerate the past in order to impress others.

Munchausen's syndrome

Munchausen's syndrome is a variant of pathological lying in which the individual presents to hospitals with bogus illnesses, complex medical histories and often multiple surgical scars. A proxy form of this condition has been described in which the individual, usually a parent, produces a factitious illness in somebody else, generally their child. This may lead to repeated presentations to hospital over a prolonged period of time and both diagnosis and management can be very challenging in these cases. The diagnosis of Munchausen's by proxy is itself a controversial diagnosis.

The role of suggestibility is important in those who present with confabulation, pseudologia, retrospective falsification or false memory. Suggestible subjects accept statements from others, act upon their commands and deny evidence from the senses or from rational understanding that would contradict these statements. Suggestibility is based either on gullibility or on implicit trust, such as that between doctor and patient. It is prominent in those who have aesthenic or hysterical personality disorders.

Vorbeireden or approximate answers

Vorbeireden or approximate answers is seen in those with hysterical pseudodementia, named after Ganser, who, in 1898 described four criminals showing several common features (Enoch *et al*, 1967). These included clouding of consciousness with disorientation, auditory and visual hallucinations (or pseudo-hallucinations), amnesia for the period during which the symptoms were manifest, conversion symptoms and recent head injury, infection or severe emotional stress. Approximate answers suggest that the patient understands the questions but appears to be deliberately avoiding the correct answer. So when asked what the capital of England is, the reply might be 'Bristol', or when asked how many eyes a dog has, the answer given is '3'. Ganser believed it to be a hysterical condition with the unconscious production of symptoms to avoid a court appearance. Some authorities reserve the term Ganser syndrome for those who have clouding of consciousness along with the other symptoms, and distinguish it from

61

pseudodementia in which consciousness is clear (Whitlock, 1967). Many now believe that the Ganser syndrome is indicative of either an organic or a psychotic state rather than hysteria as originally believed. A similar condition of approximate answers is found in those consciously feigning illness and this should be called malingering or factitious disorder according to the nature of the gain. Ganser syndrome and malingering/factitious disorder are often confused in spite of the conscious basis for the latter. *Vorbeireden* is also found in acute schizophrenia, usually the hebephrenic type.

Cryptamnesia

Cryptamnesia is described by Sims (1997) as 'the experience of not remembering that one is remembering'. For example a person writes a witty passage and does not realise that they are quoting from some passage they have seen elsewhere rather than writing something original. There is no indication as to whether this is a common phenomenon or whether it is associated with any specific psychiatric disorder.

Retrospective delusions

Retrospective delusions are found in some patients with psychoses who backdate their delusions in spite of the clear evidence that the illness is of recent origin. Thus, the person will say that they have always been persecuted or that they have always been evil. Primary delusional experiences may take the form of memories and these are known as delusional memories, consisting of sudden delusional ideas and delusional perceptions (see p. 40). Delusional memories are variously defined, some authorities believing them to be delusional interpretations of real memories (Pawar & Spence, 2003), while others, such as the Present State Examination (PSE), suggest that they are experiences of past events that did not occur but which the subject clearly 'remembers'. There are two components to a delusional memory, i.e. the perception (either real or imagined) and the memory.

Distortions of recognition

Déjà vu is not strictly a disturbance of memory, but a problem with the familiarity of places and events. It comprises the feeling of having experienced a current event in the past, although it has no basis in fact. The converse, *jamais vous* is the knowledge that an event has been experienced before but is not presently associated with the appropriate feelings of familiarity. *Déjà entendu*, the feeling of auditory recognition, and *déjà pense*, a new thought recognised as having previously occurred, are related to *déjà vu*, being different only in the modality of experience. These can be experienced by normal subjects as well as among those with temporal lobe epilepsy.

False reconnaissance is defined as false recognition or misidentification and it can occur in organic psychoses and in acute and chronic schizophrenia. It may be positive when the patient recognises strangers as their friends and relatives. In confusional states and acute schizophrenia, at most, a few people are positively misidentified. However, some chronic schizophrenics give a false identity to every person they meet. In negative misidentification the patient insists that friends and relatives are not whom they say they are and that they are strangers in disguise. Some patients assert that some or all people are doubles of the real people whom they claim to be. This is known as Capgras syndrome and occurs in schizophrenia and in dementia.

Hyperamnesia

The opposite of amnesia and paramnesia can also occur and is termed hyperamnesia, or exaggerated registration, retention and recall. Flashbulb memories are those memories that are associated with intense emotion. They are unusually vivid, detailed and long-lasting; for example many people can recall where and what they were doing when they heard the news of the death of Diana, Princess of Wales. Flashbacks are sudden intrusive memories that are associated with the cognitive and emotional experiences of a traumatic event such as an accident. It may lead to acting and/or feeling that the event is recurring and attempts have been made to use this as a defence in some murder trials. It is regarded as one of the characteristic symptoms of post-traumatic stress disorder but is also associated with substance misuse disorders and emotional events (McGee, 1984). It is also likely to be a term that is used inaccurately and should not be confused with intrusive recollections, which lack the emotional familiarity of flashbacks. Flashbacks involving hallucinogenic experiences can occur in association with hallucinogenic drugs and possibly cannabis use after the short-term effects have worn off. These incorporate visual distortions, false perceptions of movement in peripheral fields, flashes of colour, trails of images from moving objects, after-images and halos, as well as classical hallucinations. Eidetic images represent visual memories of almost hallucinatory vividness that are found in disorders due to substance misuse, especially hallucinogenic agents.

References

Bass, L. & Davis, E. (1988) *The Courage to Heal.* New York: Harper Row.

Battin, D. & Mahon, E. (2003) Symptom, screen memory and dream. The complexity of mental representation and disguise. *The Psychoanalytic Study of the Child,* **58,** 246–266.

Bonhoeffer, K.(1901) [Die akuten Geisteskrankheiten der Gewohnheitstrinker]. Jena: Gustav Fischer.

Brandon, S., Boakes, D., Glaser, D., *et al* (1998) Recovered memories of childhood sexual abuse: Implications for clinical practice. *British Journal of Psychiatry,* **172,** 296–307.

Brewin, C. R. & Andrews, B. (1998) Recovered memories of trauma. Phenomenology and cognitive mechanisms. *Clinical Psychology Review,* **18,** 949–970.

Enoch, M. D., Trethowan, W. H. & Barker, J. C. (1967) The Ganser Syndrome. In *Some Uncommon Syndromes* (ed. M. D. Enoch), pp. 41–55. Bristol: John Wright & Sons.

Freud, S., Breuer, J., Lockhurst, N., *et al* (1895) Reprinted in translation in 2004 as *Studies in Hysteria.* London: Penguin.

Good, M. I. (1998) Screen reconstructions: traumatic memory, conviction, and the problem of verification. *Journal of the American Psychoanalytic Association,* **46,** 149–183.

Gudjonsson, G. H. (1997) False memory syndrome and the retractors: methodological and theoretical issues. *Psychological Inquiry*, **8**, 296–299.

Gudjonsson, G. H., Kopelman, M. D. & MacKeith, J. A. C. (1999) Unreliable admissions of homicide. A case of misdiagnosis of amnesia and misuse of abreaction technique. *British Journal of Psychiatry*, **174**, 455–459.

Johnson, M. K., Hashtroudi, S. & Lindsay, D. S. (1993) Source monitoring. *Psychological Bulletin*, **114**, 3–28.

Loftus, E. F. (1993) The reality of repressed memories. *American Psychologist*, **48**, 518–537.

McGee, R. (1984) Flashbacks and memory phenomena. A comment on 'Flashback phenomena – clinical and diagnostic dilemmas'. *Journal of Nervous and Mental Diseases*, **172**, 273–278.

Pawar, A. V. & Spence, S. A. (2003) Defining thought broadcast: Semi-structured literature review.*British Journal of Psychiatry*, **183**, 287–291.

Sims, A. (1997) *Symptoms in the Mind. An Introduction to Descriptive Psychopathology*. London: Saunders.

Whitlock, F. A. (1967) The Ganser syndrome. *British Journal of Psychiatry*, **113**, 19–29.

CHAPTER 5

Disorders of emotion

It is customary to distinguish between feelings and emotions. A feeling can be defined as a positive or negative reaction to some experience or event and is the subjective experience of emotion. By contrast emotion is a stirred-up state caused by physiological changes occurring as a response to some event and which tends to maintain or abolish the causative event. The feelings may be those of depression, anxiety, fear, etc. Mood is a pervasive and sustained emotion that colours the person's perception of the world. Descriptions of mood should include intensity, duration and fluctuations as well as adjectival descriptions of the type. Affect, meaning short-lived emotion, is defined as the patient's present emotional responsiveness. It is what the doctor infers from the patient's body language including facial expression and it may or may not be congruent with mood. It is described as being within normal range, constricted, blunt or flat.

The classification and description of moods and emotion is bedeviled by the fact that the same terminology is used to describe those that are normal and appropriate (indeed their absence might be considered abnormal) and those that are so pathological as to warrant hospitalisation. Terms, such as depression, anxiety, etc., are examples of similar words being used for normal emotional reactions and for disorders requiring treatment. This failure to differentiate has serious implications, since not only does it cause linguistic confusion but it fails to distinguish the normal from the abnormal.

In this chapter, five levels of emotional reaction and expression that have clinical relevance will be described. The term normal emotional reactions will be used to describe emotional states that are the result of events and that lie within cultural and social norms. Abnormal emotional reactions are those that are understandable but excessive, while abnormal expressions of emotion refer to emotional expressions that are very different from the average normal reaction. Morbid disorders of emotional expression differ from abnormal expressions of emotion in that the person is unaware of the abnormality. Finally there will be a brief overview of morbid disorders of emotion.

Classification

Normal emotional reactions

Some emotional reactions are normal responses to events or to primary morbid psychological experiences. An example of the former is the grief reaction that follows the death of a loved one or the response of a previously healthy person to a life-threatening diagnosis. Among the latter is the understandable distress that many patients exhibit when they experience hallucinations or other psychotic symptoms. Unfortunately, in practice there has been little attempt to distinguish these understandable and non-morbid reactions from those that are abnormal. One problem is that many of the symptoms complained of are present both in the normal responses and in those that are abnormal; for example, following a bereavement it is expected that tearfulness, sleep disturbance, anorexia and poor concentration will occur most intensely in the initial days and will diminish over time. When the grief reaction is prolonged or becomes a depressive episode a similar constellation of symptoms is also present.

A further aspect of the distinction that has not been examined is functional incapacity, which is present in abnormal states but absent or brief in the normal reactions. Thus, the person exhibiting a normal reaction to a stressful event is unlikely to be incapacitated from carrying out their normal duties and acting in their usual roles for other than the briefest of periods. For example, how long can a person be expected to require time off work following bereavement or following a diagnosis of cancer in a spouse or child and yet be considered to be experiencing a normal reaction? There is little to assist the clinician in this regard, although a period of 6–12 months is usually mentioned in relation to the usual duration of normal grief reactions. The period of dysfunction requiring leave from work in the immediate aftermath is less certain, and probably ranges from a few days to a few weeks, though it may be influenced by other factors, such as the presence of support and practical help in such circumstances.

Abnormal emotional reactions

These are states that are understandable in the context of stressful events but are associated with more prolonged impairment in functioning. A clear representation of the distinction between normal and abnormal emotional states is illustrated by the Yerkes–Dodson curve (1908), which shows that up to a certain level of stress there is no impairment but beyond a certain point functioning deteriorates. The point at which this happens is determined by individual attributes such as genetic and personality predisposition and by external factors including social support and the duration and severity of the stressors. Diagnostically, both the *ICD–10 Classification of Mental and Behavioural Disorders* (World Health Organization, 1992) and the *Diagnostic and Statistical Manual of Mental Disorders* (American Psychiatric Association, 1994) define these abnormal emotional reactions as adjustment disorders with disturbance of mood (to include anxiety, depression, other emotions or disturbance of conduct).

Anxiety is an unpleasant affective state and a simple definition is fear for no adequate reason. Descriptive terms such as tension, stress and 'taut like a wire' are often used by the patient. Sometimes the anxiety is accompanied by physical symptoms such as palpitations, sweating, difficulty breathing, dizziness, etc., and if the physical symptoms occur suddenly, and in combination, the result is overwhelming fear, and the term panic attack is used. Anxiety may be associated with anxious foreboding, i.e. a sense that something terrible will happen but without the knowledge of what this will be. Patients often use the word anxiety to describe worry or, if asked directly if they are anxious, they may reply 'I have nothing to be anxious about'. Some of these patients, however, may admit on further questioning that they feel frightened for no reason, while others do not make the connection between the cause and their symptom. Overwhelming panic may lead to inactivity (being 'paralysed with fear') or ill-directed, chaotic over-activity.

When the fear is restricted to one object, situation or idea, the term phobia is used. Phobias are associated with physical symptoms of anxiety and with avoidance. Most fears are learned responses, such as the person who develops a fear of dogs after being bitten. Some phobias are secondary to morbid states, most commonly depressive illness, and others, such as fear of contamination, are regarded as obsessional symptoms.

Depressed mood is one of the commonly experienced abnormal reactions. Unfortunately discussion about mood is bedevilled by the use of similar words to describe different mood states (Casey *et al*, 2001). 'Depression' is a case in point, in which the term is used to describe the appropriate sadness that is associated with bereavement, the low mood that comes from frustration and the profound gloom that is part of severe depressive illness. A further complication is that depression can be a symptom secondary to another morbid process, an understandable reaction or an illness in itself.

Reactivity of mood is the term used to describe the fluctuations in mood that occur in parallel with change to one's environment. Thus mood will improve on going on holiday or when the stressful situation alters, for example difficulties with a workmate resolving when that person resigns, only to recur when re-exposed to the stressful situation. Sometimes over time there is an adaptation to the adverse conditions and the symptoms and impairment in functioning gradually improve. Sometimes there is anger and blame directed at the guilty party or situation; there may also be threats of self-harm and sleep may be disturbed.

Anxious foreboding is defined as a fear that something terrible will happen although the person cannot identify what they are frightened of. It is accompanied by physical symptoms of anxiety and must be distinguished from understandable foreboding such as experienced by a person with cancer awaiting a scan result. Anxious foreboding is present in several disorders such as generalised anxiety, depressive illness and panic disorder.

The moods experienced in these reactions do not differ qualitatively from those experienced in normal emotional reactions, in adjustment disorders, in generalised anxiety or in depressive episodes.

Abnormal expressions of emotion

These refer to emotional expressions that are very different from the average normal reaction. Those with abnormal expressions of emotion are generally aware of the abnormality. Excessive emotional response may be the result of learning and of different cultural norms. So the distraught woman screaming at the death of a loved one may be reflecting a cultural variant of normal grief.

The converse or lack of emotional response is also of great interest. Some depressed people fail to exhibit any emotion where some would be expected. For example, the person exposed to extreme stress may fail to show any emotion; this is termed 'dissociation of affect' and is said to be an unconscious defence against the impact of overwhelming stress. It may be described as a feeling of numbness. Derealisation and depersonalisation, although not primarily disorders of emotion but disorders of the experience of self, are associated with a feeling of being cut off or a feeling that objects seem distant. The accompanying feeling of being unresponsive is probably the most common example of dissociation of affect. David Livingstone the explorer wrote of this when he described the feeling he had on being seized by a lion 'It caused a sense of dreaminess in which there was no sense of pain nor feeling of terror, though I was quite conscious of all that was happening'.

An unusual but significant abnormality in the expression of emotion is that seen in the 'smiling depressive' who retains the communicatory smile but loses the emotional element. So although able to visibly smile, their eyes remain unchanged and display a tension in the surrounding muscles. This is a feature of severe depression and can beguile the unwary into underestimating the depth of the depression.

Another variant of dissociation of affect is the *belle indifférence* that is seen in conversion disorder. Although this phenomenon is rare nowadays, there are examples in the older psychiatric literature of people with gross conversion symptoms and severe disabilities who were undisturbed by their suffering. Dissociation of affect should not be applied to the emotional indifference that is often found in violent criminals, who are usually able to discuss their unpleasant crimes without any emotion.

A defence that may manifest as lack of emotion is denial. This occurs when the person denies awareness of an event even though such an event has clearly taken place, as for instance when a person is given bad news about an illness but continues as if nothing had happened and without displaying any emotion. Unfortunately the term denial is often used erroneously to describe the conscious refusal to acknowledge what is known to be true, for example that a loved one has a serious illness.

Apathy may be erroneously confused with dissociation of affect. Apathy is often used to mean emotional indifference, often with a sense of futility. It may manifest itself as a lack of motivation and is found in those in prisons, in socially deprived areas and in disorders such as schizophrenia and the amotivational syndrome associated with cannabis misuse. The former may be accompanied by blunting and/or flattening of affect.

Perplexity is a tentative or bewildered, slightly puzzled state that occurs in anxiety, mild clouding of consciousness and emerging schizophrenia, as new psychotic experiences are occurring.

Morbid expressions of emotion

This group differs from abnormal expressions of emotion (as discussed above) in that the patient is unaware of the morbidity in emotional expression even though it is apparent to observers. Inadequacy and incongruity of affect are characteristic of schizophrenia. In some patients with schizophrenia there seems to be a complete loss of all emotional life so that the patient is indifferent to their own well-being and that of others. It shows itself as insensitivity to the subtleties of social intercourse and is known as inadequacy or blunting of affect and was called 'parathymia' by Bleuler. It manifests itself as social awkwardness and inappropriateness, for example the patient who took visitors to the yard in his house to show them a dead dog. In others there seems to be a misdirection of emotions, known as incongruity, so that an indifferent event may produce a severe emotional outburst, while an event that objectively seems to be emotionally charged has no effect on the patient's emotional response. Some argue that this may not necessarily be a primary disorder of affect but a congruous response to the distorted environment associated with delusions and other psychotic phenomena experienced by the patient with schizophrenia. Finally, emotional constriction and its more severe form, flattening, are evident by a limitation in the usual range of emotional responses so that that the patient displays little emotional response in any direction, although that which is expressed is in the appropriate direction, unlike incongruity of affect, which is not. Some patients with chronic schizophrenia describe a complicated system of paranoid delusions with very little emotion, clearly showing flattening of affect. Others, however, describe grandiose delusions with much enthusiasm or paranoid delusions with great anger and bitterness; if they are depressed or elated this may overshadow an underlying flattening, but it may also be evidence of appropriate affect. Stiffening of affect may also be seen in some patients with schizophrenia when their emotional response is at first congruent but does not alter as the situation changes.

Incongruity of affect should not be confused with the embarrassed smile of the anxious person recounting a painful or embarrassing topic. Some patients with depression also smile and this may be mistaken for incongruity of affect or it may even mask the low mood, in the past called 'masked' or 'smiling' depression. Smiling is normally an expression of cheerfulness, contentment or well-being but it has an important function in communication between people. There are also the smiles that indicate friendliness, smiles that ask for help and there is the placatory smile. Psychiatrists should be able to distinguish between these smiles and the communicatory smile of the depressed person. Unless the person is overwhelmed by their miseries they can produce this – a smile that may be trying to conceal sadness or that may be trying to say 'Don't worry about me; I'm all right'. Psychiatrists should not be deceived by the smile, as it may lead to an underestimation of the degree of depression. This is particularly important when assessing suicide risk. The experienced observer will notice that the depressed person smiles with the lips and not the eyes, so that despite their apparent cheerfulness there is a hardness and lack of movement of the muscles around the eyes. Whenever a patient has morbid ideas of a depressive kind and appears to be fairly cheerful, the doctor should probe carefully into the most sensitive areas of the patient's life and watch for the emergence of depression. Expressions of empathy and support may also evoke an emotional reaction that allows the underlying depression to manifest itself. Those in mixed states may also smile excessively, while concealing depression, but this is usually temporary with the mood appearing to be labile and fluctuating rather than fixed.

Lability of affect is found in many conditions. It is defined as rapid and abrupt changes in emotion largely unrelated to external stimuli. These shifts occur without warning. It is found in some people with no psychiatric disorder. For example, those who are very soft-hearted may be easily moved to tears. Those with personality disorder of the borderline type may also exhibit lability of affect. However, it is most common in mixed affective states (dysphoric mania) and in mania where short bursts of weeping are present. It may also be a feature in organic brain disease following damage to the frontal lobe or following cerebrovascular accidents. Patients with depressive illness may have difficulty controlling their emotions, so that distressing events that normally would produce a transient feeling of unhappiness may cause them to cry and they are often made worse by sympathy.

In emotional lability patients have difficulty controlling their emotions, but in affective incontinence there is total loss of control and this is particularly common in cerebral atherosclerosis and in multiple sclerosis, where spontaneous outbursts of laughter or crying occur. In its most severe form the terms 'forced laughing' and 'forced weeping' are used to describe this, but there is a mismatch between the emotional expression and the subjective feelings since there is an absence of concomitant feelings of happiness or sadness.

Morbid disorders of emotion

These can be regarded as pathological states that, although sometimes triggered by stressful events, do not spontaneously resolve with removal of the stressor, as in adjustment disorders, and therefore have their own independent momentum. These also include those states that arise without any precipitant. These are classified in ICD–10 and DSM–IV (see also Chapter 1). Depressive illness is the most common in this group and qualitative differences between this mood state and the understandably low mood that is secondary to, say, bereavement, are described by many patients who can distinguish their understandable reactions to stressors from the pathologically low mood that is depressive illness. None the less, it is difficult scientifically to demonstrate these differences as the neurobiology underpinning this subjective distinction has yet to be verified.

Those with depressive illness use terms such as 'a weight', 'a cloud' or 'a darkness' to attempt to capture the exact emotional feeling. The morbid sadness in this illness may be associated with morbid thinking that may reach delusional intensity. The delusions in morbid depression have already been discussed (see pp. 44–46.). Often there is inhibition of thinking, loss of drive and decreased voluntary activity. The physical and/or psychological slowing that occurs is known as psychomotor retardation. There may be difficulty making decisions due either to poor concentration or to obsessional doubting, secondary to the mood state. Inner unrest, loss of confidence, anxiety and an inability to enjoy anything in life or even get pleasure from everyday occurrences (anhedonia), for example being hugged by one's children, a fine spring morning, etc., are prominent. Anhedonia, a term coined in 1896 by Ribot, a French psychologist (Nicolas & Murray, 1999), is a core symptom in depressive illness. As Hamlet said

'How weary, stale flat, and unprofitable
Seem to me all the uses of this world'.

All experiences are considered from the worst aspect and everything is seen in a gloomy light. Only troubling thoughts, often with the same content, spontaneously come into the mind, so that the patient is very frequently preoccupied by unpleasant thoughts and has difficulty in thinking. Often the patient feels a tight band around his head and there may be a sense of oppression in the chest associated with anxiety, for which Schneider used the term 'vital hypochondriacal depression'. A related and more modern concept is somatisation, or the presence of somatic features, in which there is misattribution of symptoms as due to physical illness rather than having a psychiatric cause. This is often corrected with education, when a new insight is reached regarding the physical symptoms.

Morbid depression also abolishes the normal reactive changes of emotion or emotional resonance. This leads to a sense of inner emptiness or deadness, so the patient does not feel they are participating in the world any more. This loss of feeling for the environment gives the person with depression the impression of unreality. This loss of emotional resonance gives rise to complaints of depersonalisation and derealisation in morbid depression but is obviously not at all the same. Possibly this mechanism is partly responsible for depersonalisation in schizophrenia but here the symptom appears to result more from the subjective experience of the breakdown of the boundaries of the self, which finally become obvious in apophanous experiences, passivity feelings and thought alienation.

Morbid depression is usually associated with diurnal variation in mood or in other symptoms such as anxiety, loss of energy and libido, anorexia and early morning wakening, but initial or middle insomnia are also described. If depression is severe and psychomotor retardation is marked, depressive stupor may occur. The apparent indifference of the person with severe depression must be differentiated from the apathy and lack of concern of the person with schizophrenia. While the person with schizophrenia does not care that housework is left undone, the person with severe depression is able to understand its necessity but is unable to act and experiences their failure to do so with shame and guilt.

Apart from depressive illness and bipolar disorder, morbid depression is also found in schizophrenia and in acute and chronic organic states. Sometimes the depressed mood may be secondary to insight in the schizophrenic process or into the likely consequences of failing memory, while in others it is an integral part of the process itself.

Morbid anxiety frequently occurs in association with morbid depression and can cause difficulties in diagnosing depression. In severe form it can present a picture of agitation. However, there is no one-to-one relationship between the inner psychic feeling of anxiety and the external manifestation of agitation. Morbid anxiety is also found in organic states and may sometimes be secondary to terrifying visual hallucinations. Acute and chronic brain disease, when mild, can produce anxiety mixed with depression and irritability. This was previously called 'organic neurasthenia'. Anxiety and fear are often present in psychotic states such as paranoid schizophrenia but this may not be morbid but rather a natural reaction to delusions and hallucinations.

Irritability may be seen in depressive illness and schizophrenia. In depression and schizophrenia this may be an exaggeration of underlying personality attributes, although not inevitably so. In mania or hypomania the patient is often cheerful and elated but there is frequently significant irritability also. Irritability is also prominent in mixed states in which the patient is both depressed and manic/hypomanic simultaneously (known as dysphoric mania). Short-lived periods of depression, euphoria, anxiety or unpleasant feelings lasting no longer than a few minutes may be symptomatic of temporal lobe foci.

Extreme apathy may be a feature of severe depression, schizophrenia or damage to the frontal lobe. Morbid euphoria and elation classically occur in mania and hypomania but can also be seen in organic states and in schizophrenia, especially the hebephrenic subtype, where the patient presents as silly and annoying. In mania and hypomania the elation is not related to any specific event and is not modified by depressing influences. In both there is an increased pressure of speech with prolixity, and flight of ideas or a subjective awareness of racing thoughts (see p. 34–35). Superficial bustling activity, disinhibition, distractibility, sometimes hypersexuality and a tendency to be argumentative if thwarted are also present. Many projects may be initiated but none completed. In milder forms, the pathological nature of the condition may not be apparent to family or friends. Instead it may be felt that the person is just a 'cheerful sort' or good fun, and the associated symptoms may appear relatively mild, but eventually these may lead to faulty judgement and some overactivity; often it is only then that the pathological basis for the behaviour becomes apparent. Sometimes the patient feels distinctly unwell, restless and out-of-control, and seeks help themselves. The distinction between mania and hypomania lies in the presence of psychotic symptoms in the former, typically grandiose delusions, and/or 'marked' impairment in functioning; DSM−IV, however, does not provide any definition of 'marked'. The addition of bipolar II disorder to DSM−IV in 1994 occurred in response to the increasing evidence that milder forms of illness, besides classic manic−depression (bipolar I) could also occur and remain undiagnosed. This has opened the debate in recent years concerning bipolar spectrum disorder and the upper and lower borders on this continuum, with some suggesting that up to four levels of bipolar disorder exist along this spectrum (Akiskal & Pinto, 1999) and that many diagnoses of agitated depression may in fact be variants of bipolar spectrum disorder, with all that this implies for treatment.

Lesions of the hypothalamus may produce a clinical picture resembling mania with flight of ideas. Euphoria also occurs in multiple sclerosis, when it is associated with a sense of well-being and is linked to the degree of organic brain change (Benedict *et al*, 2004). Euphoria and a passive attitude may also feature in the amnestic syndrome and in lesions of the frontal lobe. Frontal-lobe damage with euphoria, often presenting as silliness, lack of foresight and indifference, is known as moria or *Witzelsucht*.

Ecstasy is an exalted state of feeling and is therefore different from the morbid cheerful mood or elation. It can occur in the healthy population at times of profound religious experience or occasions of deep emotion such as following childbirth. The psychiatrist is interested when this state is abnormal in degree so that self-neglect or neglect of others is present, or when it is prolonged. It is a state of extreme well-being associated with a feeling of rapture, bliss and grace. Unlike elation, it is not associated with overactivity or flight of ideas. The mind is usually occupied with a feeling of communion with God or some religious figure. There may be a feeling of being in tune with the whole of nature and at one with the universe. Sometimes it may be associated with grandiose delusions, as when, for example, a patient with schizophrenia sat smiling to himself and when asked why declared that he was the King of Israel and was about to marry the Queen of Heaven. Ecstatic states may occur in schizophrenia, in those who misuse lysergic acid diethylamide, in epilepsy and in mass hysteria associated with religious services. In the last it begins in a single individual and spreads thereafter. Unlike the person experiencing passivity phenomena, the person in ecstasy experiences the change in ego boundaries as voluntary and lacking the interference associated with the former (Sims, 2003). Time may be experienced as standing still.

References

Akiskal, H. S. & Pinto, O. (1999) The evolving bipolar spectrum. Prototypes I,II,III and IV. *Psychiatric Clinics of North America*, **22**, 517−534.

American Psychiatric Association (1994) *Diagnostic and Statistical Manual of Mental Disorders* (4th edn) (DSM−IV). Washington, DC: APA.

Benedict, R. H., Carone, D. A. & Bakshi, R. (2004) Correlating brain atrophy with cognitive dysfunction, mood disturbances, and personality disorder in multiple sclerosis. *Journal of Neuroimaging*, **14** (suppl. 3), 36−45.

Casey, P., Dowrick, C. & Wilkinson, G. (2001) Adjustment disorders: fault line in the psychiatric glossary. *British Journal of Psychaitry*, **179**, 479−481.

Nicolas, S. & Murray, D. J. (1999) Theodule Ribot (1839−1916), founder of French psychology: A biographical introduction. *History of Psychology*, **2**, 161−169.

Sims, A. (2003) *Symptoms in the Mind. An Introduction to Descriptive Psychopathology* (3rd edn). London: Saunders.

World Health Organization (1992) *The ICD–10 Classification of Mental and Behavioural Disorders: Clinical Descriptions and Diagnostic Guidelines* (10th edn). Geneva: WHO.

Yerkes, R. H. & Dodson, J. D. (1908) The relation of strength of stimulus to rapidity of habit formation. *Journal of Comparative Neurological Psychology*, **18**, 459−482.

CHAPTER 6

Disorders of the experience of self

Recent decades have seen a revival of interest in the study of the self, self-awareness and various changes in self-awareness, especially in the context of mental illnesses such as schizophrenia (Sass & Parnas, 2003; Harland et al, 2004). Although there is a substantial German literature on *Ichbewusstsein* or ego consciousness, both of these terms have now been replaced by the term 'self-experience.' Jaspers (1997) has pointed out that there are four aspects of self-experience, the awareness of:

- existence and activity of the self
- being a unity at any given point in time
- continuity of identity over a period of time
- being separate from the environment (or, in other words, awareness of ego boundaries).

It is possible to discuss disorders of self-awareness under these four headings, but a number of other symptoms can be regarded as disturbances in two of these aspects of self-experience: awareness of existence and activity of the self and awareness of being separate from the environment.

Disturbance of awareness of self-activity

All events that can be brought into consciousness are associated with a sense of personal possession, although this is not usually in the forefront of consciousness. This 'I' quality has been called personalisation (Jaspers, 1997) and may be disturbed in psychological disorders. There are two aspects to the sense of self-activity: the sense of existence and the awareness of the performance of one's actions.

Depersonalisation

A change in the awareness of one's own activity occurs when the patient feels that they are no longer their normal natural self and this is known as 'depersonalisation'. Often this is associated with a feeling of unreality so that the environment is experienced as flat, dull and unreal. This aspect of the symptom is known as 'derealisation'. The feeling of unreality is the core of this symptom, and it is always, to a greater or lesser extent, an unpleasant experience; which distinguishes it from ecstatic states.

When the patient first experiences the symptom they are likely to find it very frightening and often think it is a sign that they are going mad. In the course of time they may become more or less accustomed to it. Many patients who complain of depersonalisation also state that their capacity for feeling is diminished or absent. This is a subjective experience because to the outside observer there is no loss of ability to respond emotionally and appropriately to any given situation. It is important to remember that depersonalisation is not a delusion and it should be distinguished from nihilistic delusions in which the patient denies that they exist or that they are alive, or that the world or other people exist.

The *ICD−10 Classification of Mental and Behavioural Disorders* (ICD−10; World Health Organization, 1992) provides a clinical description of depersonalisation−derealisation syndrome and lists diagnostic criteria that include depersonalisation and derealisation symptoms occurring in a setting of clear consciousness, with retention of insight. The *Diagnostic and Statistical Manual of Mental Disorders* (DSM−IV; American Psychiatric Association, 1994) provides a clinical description of depersonalisation disorder that emphasises recurrent feelings of detachment, retention of reality-testing, and resultant personal distress, all occurring in the absence of another mental disorder. While the epidemiology of depersonalisation disorder remains poorly understood, it is thought to be twice as common in women as in men (Kaplan & Saddock, 1996).

An emotional crisis or a threat to life may lead to complete dissociation of affect, which can be regarded as an adaptive mechanism that allows the subject to function reasonably without being overwhelmed by emotion. Milder degrees of dissociative depersonalisation occur in moderately stressful situations, so that depersonalisation is quite a common experience and is reported to occur at least once in 30−70% of young adults (Freeman, 1996).

Since dissociative depersonalisation appears to be a relatively common experience, some patients may complain of dissociation when they realise that it is a symptom in which doctors are interested. This may explain the increase in complaints of depersonalisation seen among patients in a 'neurosis unit' following the admission of a patient with hysterical depersonalisation.

Depersonalisation may also be reported in association with schizophrenia, depressive illness, organic brain disease or substance misuse (for example, lysergic acid diethylamide) (Sims, 1995; Freeman, 1996). Very occasionally, depersonalisation may be the outstanding feature in a patient with a depressive state. This may give rise to a mistaken diagnosis of schizophrenia because the patient may have great difficulty in describing depersonalisation and the examiner may be misled by the bizarre description of the symptom.

It should also be noted that delusions of nihilism are sometimes described as delusions of depersonalisation; in most of these cases, mental state examination will readily reveal that these are mood-congruent delusions occurring in the setting of severe depression. Depersonalisation and related phenomena may also occur from time to time in individuals without mental illness, especially when severely tired.

Loss of emotional resonance

In depression there is not only a general lowering of mood, but there is a loss of the normal emotional resonance. Normally everyone experiences a series of positive and negative feelings as they encounter both animate and inanimate objects in the environment. In depression this natural emotional resonance may be absent and the patient has the feeling that they cannot feel. This lack of natural feeling is usually most marked when the patient with depression encounters their loved ones. If the patient has ideas of guilt, this apparent loss of feeling will make the patient feel even more guilty and morally reprehensible. There may be similar loss of emotional resonance in certain other conditions apart from depression, including, for example, depersonalisation states (see above).

Disturbances in the immediate awareness of self-unity

In psychogenic and depressive depersonalisation the patient may feel that they are talking and acting in an automatic way. This may lead them to say that they feel 'as if' they are two persons. Individuals with appreciation-needing personalities or with learning disability may leave out the 'as if' and say that they are two people. A patient with certain delusions (for example, delusions of demoniac possession) may also feel that they are two people (for example themselves and the Devil). In addition, patients with schizophrenia may feel they are two or more people, although this is not common.

Disturbance of the continuity of self

Individuals with schizophrenia may feel that they are not the same person that they were before the illness. This may be expressed as a sense of change, but some patients may claim that they died under their old name and have come to life as a new person. This sense of complete change of the personality may be described in the context of religious conversion and some individuals may refer to this as 'being born again'.

Very rarely, patients may complain of experiencing multiple different personalities. The ICD−10 provides a clinical description of multiple personality disorder in the category of dissociative and conversion disorders, and emphasises that this disorder is both rare and controversial. The DSM−IV includes diagnostic criteria for dissociative identity disorder (which includes what is commonly known as multiple personality disorder), and emphasises the disorder's strong association with traumatic events, such as childhood sexual abuse. The differential diagnosis includes other dissociative disorders, schizophrenia, rapid-cycling bipolar disorder, borderline personality disorder, malingering and complex partial epilepsy.

Some individuals with schizophrenia, following an acute shift of the illness, may describe how they seemed to pass from being one personality to being another. Others may describe how they seemed to be personifying natural events, animals and historical figures during the acute illness.

Disturbances of the boundaries of the self

One of the most fundamental of experiences is the difference between one's body and the rest of the world. Some psychoanalysts have suggested that this distinction is acquired in later life and that the young infant is unable to differentiate between itself and the rest of the world. The distinction between what pertains to one's body and what does not is, in fact, largely attributable to the function of the proprioceptive system. Knowledge of what is the body and what is not is based on the link between information from the exteroceptors and the proprioceptors, a link that is probably learned and has to be maintained constantly.

This can be readily demonstrated; anybody who has had a finger anaesthetised knows that when touched it feels like a foreign object, i.e. not part of the body. The same phenomenon occurs when the local anaesthetic for a dental operation produces anaesthesia of the lip. Equally relevant to this is the experience of patients who have lesions of the brain that give rise to disturbances of body image. The physiological schema of the body and the continuity and integrity of memory and psychological function is the basis for the awareness of the 'self'.

Disturbances of body image occur in a range of conditions, including hypnagogic states, depression, schizophrenia and organic disorders. On the occasions when a depressed individual states that their face has become ugly, this statement may need to be interpreted in a metaphorical sense, with due regard to the prevailing mood state.

Many symptoms of schizophrenia can be seen as aspects of a breakdown of the boundary between self and the environment. In the early stages of acute schizophrenia, the individual may experience this breakdown of the limits of them self as a change in their awareness of their own activity that is becoming alienated from them. This is probably not the same as that which occurs in some patients with depersonalisation who say that they feel like machines, as if their actions were carried out automatically. 'Loss of control' may also be reported in obsessions and compulsions, where the thought or impulse to action is experienced as belonging to the patient but occurring against their wishes.

In the alienation of personal action that occurs in schizophrenia, the patient has the experience that their actions are under the control of some external power. Alienation of thought has already been discussed in the section on disorders of thinking, but the alienation may affect motor actions and feelings, in which case it is customary to use the term 'passivity phenomena.' The patient 'knows' that their actions are not their own, and may attribute this control to hypnosis, radio waves, the internet, and so on. One patient expressed his passivity feelings by saying 'I am a guided missile.' This patient experienced penile erections during the night that he 'knew' were produced by the night nurse influencing him with her thoughts as she sat at her desk some 20 feet away. These phenomena have also been described as 'made' or 'fabricated' experiences because the patient experiences these phenomena as being made by an outside influence. The term 'made experience' is also used for 'apophanous experience', when the patient knows that all the events around them are being made for their benefit; this symptom has been particularly associated with schizophrenia, once organic brain disorders have been excluded.

Another aspect of the loss of the boundary with the environment is seen when the patient 'knows' that their actions and thoughts have excessive effect on the world around them, and he experiences activity that is not directly related to them as having an effect on them. For example, a patient may believe that when they pass urine, they cause bad things to happen to other people. Thought broadcasting, which we have previously discussed as a variety of thought alienation, can also be regarded as the result of the breakdown of ego boundaries, because the patient 'knows' that as he thinks the whole world is thinking in unison.

Theory of mind, consciousness and schizophrenia

Many of these disturbances in the experience of self may coexist with deficits in the patient's ability to understand the psychological states of other people, especially in the context of psychosis. The term 'theory of mind' specifically refers to the ability of an individual to infer or understand the mental states of others in given situations; this is also known as mentalisation (for an overview of theory of mind in relation to psychosis, see Bentall, 2003). Deficits in theory of mind have been particularly associated with autism (Baron-Cohen et al, 1993) and also with paranoid symptoms in psychotic illnesses (Frith, 1992; Frith & Corcoran, 1996). While there is now evidence that theory-of-mind deficits are unlikely to be specific to paranoia (Langdon et al, 1997) and are not invariably present in schizophrenia (McCabe et al, 2004), this approach may none the less prove valuable in informing other approaches to understanding the psychopathology of schizophrenia (Bentall, 2003) or elucidating aetiology. Schiffman et al (2004), for example, recently reported significant evidence of deficits in perspective-taking among children who went on later to develop schizophrenia spectrum disorders, suggesting that some aspect of theory of mind may be impaired in these individuals prior to the development of these disorders.

Sass & Parnas (2003) have proposed a unified account of symptoms in schizophrenia, in which they emphasised the importance of underlying abnormalities of consciousness and argued that schizophrenia is fundamentally a self-disorder characterised by particular distortions of awareness of aspects of the self (for example, increased self-consciousness, diminished self-affection). The study of consciousness and the study of theory of mind are clearly related fields within schizophrenia research, and the current balance of evidence suggests that while the precise nature of disturbances in these domains is not yet clear, they may well play an important role in determining the clinical features of the illness. The next chapter is devoted to the disturbances of consciousness that are commonly seen in mental illness.

References

American Psychiatric Association (1994) *Diagnostic and Statistical Manual of Mental Disorders* (DSM–IV). Washington, DC: APA.

Baron-Cohen, S., Tager-Flusberg, H. & Cohen, D. J. (1993) *Understanding Other Minds: Perspectives from Autism.* Oxford: Oxford University Press.

Bentall, R. P. (2003) *Madness Explained: Psychosis and Human Nature.* London: Allen Lane.

Freeman, C. P. L. (1996) Neurotic disorders. In *Companion to Psychiatric Studies* (5th edn) (eds R. E. Kendell & A. K. Zealley). Edinburgh: Churchill Livingstone.

Frith, C. D. (1992) *The Cognitive Neuropsychology of Schizophrenia.* Hillsdale, NJ: Lawrence Erlbaum.

Frith, C. D. & Corcoran, R. (1996) Exploring 'theory of mind' in people with schizophrenia. *Psychological Medicine,* **26,** 521–530.

Harland, R., Morgan, C. & Hutchinson, G. (2004) Phenomenology, science and the anthropology of the self: a new model for the aetiology of psychosis. *British Journal of Psychiatry,* **185,** 361–362.

Jaspers, K. (1997) *General Psychopathology* (trans. J. Hoenig & M. W. Hamilton). Baltimore: Johns Hopkins University Press.

Kaplan, H. I. & Saddock, B. J. (1996) *Concise Textbook of Clinical Psychiatry* (7th edn). Baltimore: Williams & Wilkins.

Langdon, R., Michie, P., Ward, P. B., *et al* (1997) Defective self and/or other mentalizing in schizophrenia: a cognitive neuropsychological approach. *Cognitive Neuropsychiatry,* **2,** 167–193.

McCabe, R., Leudar, I. & Antaki, C. (2004) Do people with schizophrenia display theory of mind deficits in clinical interactions? *Psychological Medicine,* **34,** 401–412.

Sass, L. A. & Parnas, J. (2003) Schizophrenia, consciousness and the self. *Schizophrenia Bulletin,* **29,** 427–444.

Schiffman, J., Lam, C. W., Jiwatram, T., *et al* (2004) Perspective-taking deficits in people with schizophrenia spectrum disorders: a prospective investigation. *Psychological Medicine,* **34,** 1581–1586.

Sims, A. (1995) *Symptoms in the Mind: An Introduction to Descriptive Psychopathology* (2nd edn). London: Saunders.

World Health Organization (1992). *The ICD–10 Classification of Mental and Behavioural Disorders: Clinical Descriptions and Diagnostic Guidelines* (10th edn). Geneva: WHO.

Disorders of consciousness

Recent decades have seen a considerable renaissance of scientific interest in the study of human consciousness in general (Edelman, 1989; Dennett, 1991; Damasio, 2000). For the purposes of descriptive clinical psychopathology, consciousness can be simply defined as a state of awareness of the self and the environment. In the fully awake subject the intensity of consciousness varies considerably. If someone is carrying out a difficult experiment their level of consciousness will be at its height, but when they are sitting in an armchair glancing though the newspaper the intensity of their consciousness will be much less. In fact, when subjects are monitoring a monotonously repetitive set of signals, short periods of sleep may occur between signals and are not recognised by the subject, but are shown clearly by changes in the electroencephalogram (EEG).

Before we can discuss the disorders of consciousness we must deal with the possibly confounding issue of attention. Attention can be active when the subject focuses their attention on some internal or external event, or passive when the same events attract the subject's attention without any conscious effort on their part. Active and passive attention are reciprocally related to each other, since the more the subject focuses their attention the greater must be the stimulus that will distract them (i.e. bring passive attention into action).

Disturbance of active attention shows itself as distractibility, so that the patient is diverted by almost all new stimuli and habituation to new stimuli takes longer than usual. It can occur in fatigue, anxiety, severe depression, mania, schizophrenia and organic states. In abnormal and morbid anxiety, active attention may be made difficult by anxious preoccupations, while in some organic states and paranoid schizophrenia, distractibility may be the result of a paranoid frame of mind. In other individuals with acute schizophrenia, distraction may be regarded as the result of formal thought disorder because the patient is unable to keep the marginal thoughts (which are connected with external objects by displacement, condensation and symbolism) out of their thinking, so that irrelevant external objects are incorporated into their thinking.

Attention is affected by an individual's mind-set, which, in the absence of mental illness, is generally non-rigid and is altered in response to incoming information. In the amnestic syndrome, however, the patient's thinking and observation are dominated by rigid sets, so that perception and comprehension are affected by selective attention.

Disorders of consciousness are associated with disorders of perception, attention, attitudes, thinking, registration and orientation. The patient with disturbance of consciousness usually shows, therefore, a discrepancy between their grasp of the environment and their social situation, personal appearance and occupation. This lack of comprehension in the absence of other florid symptoms of disordered consciousness may lead to a mistaken diagnosis of dementia. The clinical test for disturbance of consciousness is to ask the patient the date, the day of the week, the time of day, the place, the duration of their stay in that place, and so on. In other words, one tests the patient's orientation and if they are disoriented there is a prima facie case that they have an organic disorder. If this is of recent origin, then it is an acute organic state with disturbance of consciousness. Exceptions to this rule may include the patient with chronic schizophrenia, for example, who has been institutionalised on a long-term basis and may be indifferent or reject all contact, and so seem disoriented. It is important to note that patients with schizophrenia, regardless of their history of institutionalisation, may also demonstrate significant disturbances of memory (McKenna *et al*, 1990), including impairments of working and semantic memory (Kuperberg & Heckers, 2000); these impairments may also have a significant impact on social functioning.

Although disorientation in an acute illness is strongly suggestive of disordered consciousness, the absence of this sign does not rule out an acute organic state with a mild disorder of consciousness. Poor performance on intellectual and memory tasks, inability to estimate the passage of time, and changes in the EEG may all suggest an acute organic state.

Orientation is normally described in terms of time, place and person. When consciousness is disturbed it tends to affect these three aspects in that order. Orientation in time requires that an individual should maintain a continuous awareness of what goes on around them and be able to recognise the significance of those events that mark the passage of time. When the customary events that mark the passage of time are missing, it is very easy to become more or less disoriented in time. Everybody who has been away on holiday in a strange place or been in hospital for a few days has experienced this. Orientation for place is retained more easily because the surroundings provide some clues. Orientation for person is lost with greatest difficulty because the persons themselves provide the information that identifies them.

If a patient is disoriented for time and place, it is customary to say that they are confused. Unfortunately, this word is used in everyday speech to mean 'muddled', 'bewildered' or 'perplexed'. In fact, most patients with confusion are perplexed, but this sign is also seen in severe anxiety and acute schizophrenia in the absence of disorientation.

Consciousness can be changed in three basic ways: it may be dream-like, depressed or restricted.

Dream-like change of consciousness

With dream-like change of consciousness, there is some lowering of the level of consciousness, which is the subjective experience of a rise in the threshold for all incoming stimuli. The patient is disoriented for time and place, but not for person. The outstanding feature in this state is often the presence of visual hallucinations, usually of small animals and associated with fear or even terror. The patient is unable to distinguish between their mental images and perceptions, so that their mental images acquire the value of perceptions. As would be expected, thinking is disordered as it is in dreams and shows excessive displacement, condensation and misuse of symbols. Occasionally, Lilliputian hallucinations occur and are associated with a feeling of pleasure. Elementary auditory hallucinations are common, but continuous voices are rare and organised auditory hallucinations take the form of odd disconnected words or phrases. Rarely, hallucinatory voices occur in association with a dream-like change in consciousness, and if they do, the change of consciousness and the visual hallucinations often disappear in a few days, leaving behind an organic hallucinosis with little or no change in consciousness. Other hallucinations of touch, pain, electric feelings, muscle sense and vestibular sensations often occur. The patient is fearful and often misinterprets the behaviour of others as threats. Thus, a patient with delirium tremens said 'Don't hit me; please, don't hit me' whenever anyone approached, although he had never been subjected to assault. The patient is usually restless and may carry out the customary actions of this trade; this is known as 'occupational delirium'. For example, an accountant may make out a long series of accounts or a bus conductor may ask other patients for their bus fares. When the underlying physical illness is severe, insomnia is marked, and usually the disturbance of consciousness is worse at night.

So far we have been describing the acute delirium in which a dream-like change of consciousness is the outstanding feature, but milder degrees of delirium may also occur. Thus a patient may have a general lowering of consciousness during the day and be incoherent and confused. At night delirium occurs with visual hallucinations and restlessness, but it improves in the morning. Apart from a lowering of consciousness, there may also be some restriction so that the mind is dominated by a few ideas, attitudes and hallucinations. This milder type of delirium has been called a 'toxic confusional state' but this term is somewhat unsatisfactory as it is used in different senses by different practitioners. The *ICD–10 Classification of Mental and Behavioural Disorders* (ICD–10; World Health Organization,

1992) provides a more standardised terminology and clinical descriptions of a range of states of delirium, emphasising the rapid onset, fluctuating course and relatively short duration of delirium (less than 6 months), when compared to dementia. States of delirium associated with the use of psychoactive substances are classified elsewhere in ICD–10.

In the milder varieties of delirium the patient may have inconsistent orientation, so that they may be able to give their address and say that they are in hospital but insist that their home is next door, although it is really several miles away. Orientation may also vary during 24 hours of the day, so that when seen in the morning the patient may be reasonably well-orientated, but at night is utterly confused. These milder varieties of delirium may pass over into an amnestic state, torpor, severe delirium or a twilight state (see below).

Lowering of consciousness

With lowering of consciousness the patient is psychologically benumbed and there is a general lowering of consciousness without hallucinations, illusions, delusions and restlessness. The patient is apathetic, generally slowed down, unable to express themself clearly, and may perseverate. There is no accepted term for this state that is best designated as 'torpor'. In the past, this type of consciousness was very often the result of severe infections such as typhoid and typhus. Nowadays, it is more commonly seen in the context of arteriosclerotic cerebral disease following a cerebrovascular accident. If the history of the illness is not clear, the general defect in intelligence, in the absence of hallucinations, may be mistakenly diagnosed as severe dementia, but after some weeks there is a remarkable partial recovery and the patient is left with a mild organic deficit.

Restriction of consciousness

With restriction of consciousness, awareness is narrowed down to a few ideas and attitudes that dominate the patient's mind. There is some lowering of the level of consciousness, so that in some cases the patient may only appear slightly bemused and uninformed bystanders may not realise that they are confused. Disorientation for time and place occurs. Some of these patients are relatively well-ordered in their behaviour and may wander, but usually they are not able to fend for themselves, like the patient with a hysterical twilight state.

The term 'twilight state' describes conditions in which there was a restriction of the morbidly changed consciousness, a break in the continuity of consciousness, and relatively well-ordered behaviour. If one keeps strictly to these criteria, then the commonest twilight state is the result of epilepsy. However, this term has been used for any condition in which there is a real or apparent restriction of consciousness, so that simple, hallucinatory, perplexed, excited, expansive, psychomotor and orientated twilight states have been described.

The ICD–10 includes twilight states under the headings of dissociative (conversion) disorders and, when criteria for organic aetiology are met, organic mental disorders (World Health Organization, 1992). Sims (1995) notes that the term usually refers to an organic state, which is characterised by sudden onset and end, variable duration, and the occurrence of unexpected violent or emotional behaviours (Lishman, 1998).

In severe anxiety the patient may be so preoccupied by their conflicts that they are not fully aware of their environment and find that they have only a hazy idea of what has happened in the past hour or so. This may suggest to the patient that amnesia is a solution for their problems, so that they 'forget' their personal identity and the whole of their past as a temporary solution for their difficulties. This restriction of consciousness resulting from unconscious motives has been termed a 'hysterical twilight state'. It may be difficult to decide how much the motivation of a hysterical twilight state is unconscious because in some cases the subject seems to be deliberately running away from his troubles.

Wandering states with some loss of memory have also been called fugues, but not all fugues are hysterical; for example, some individuals with depression may start out to kill themselves and wander about indecisively for some days before finding their way home or being stopped by the police. Hysterical fugue may be more common in subjects who have previously had a head injury with concussion, possibly because they are familiar with the pattern of amnesia from their past experience of concussion and can therefore present it as a hysterical symptom. The ICD–10 includes dissociative fugue under the heading of dissociative (conversion) disorders and notes that conscious simulation of fugue may be difficult to differentiate from true dissociative fugue (World Health Organization, 1992). Fugue states may be of variable duration, with some fugue states persisting for extremely long periods of time.

The 1984 film *Paris, Texas* provides a vivid depiction of a man with a dissociative fugue state. Written by Sam Shepard and directed by Wim Wenders, *Paris, Texas* focuses on the story of Travis, a middle-aged man who reappears in Texas after wandering for 4 years in a desert on the border between the USA and Mexico. Despite being apparently mute and amnesic, Travis manages to locate his brother and gradually starts to re-integrate with society. The film provides a valuable demonstration of the features of dissociative fugue states, as well as a useful exploration of the difficulties that can result from them.

References

Damasio, A. (2000) *The Feeling of What Happens: Body, Emotion and the Making of Consciousness*. London: Vintage.

Dennett, D. (1991) *Consciousness Explained*. Boston: Little, Brown.

Edelman, G. (1989) *The Remembered Present*. New York: Basic Books.

Kuperberg, G. & Heckers, S. (2000) Schizophrenia and cognitive function. *Current Opinion in Neurobiology*, **10**, 205–210.

Lishman, W. A. (1998) *Organic Psychiatry: The Psychological Consequences of Cerebral Disorder* (3rd edn). Oxford: Blackwell Science.

McKenna, P. J., Tamlyn, D., Lund, C. E., *et al* (1990). Amnesic syndrome in schizophrenia. *Psychological Medicine*, **20**, 967–972.

Sims, A. (1995) *Symptoms in the Mind: An Introduction to Descriptive Psychopathology* (2nd edn). London: Saunders.

World Health Organization (1992) *The ICD–10 Classification of Mental and Behavioural Disorders: Clinical descriptions and diagnostic guidelines*. Geneva: WHO.

CHAPTER 8

Motor disorders

Psychiatric illness may be associated with objective or subjective motor disorders. This chapter is chiefly devoted to objective motor disorders. However, it is important to note at the outset that subjective motor disorders may also occur.

Subjective motor disorders: the alienation of motor acts

Normally humans experience their actions as being their own and as being under their own control, although this sense of personal control is never in the forefront of consciousness, except when a particular effort is made to overcome the effects of fatigue or toxic substances that are clouding our consciousness and making it difficult for us to control our bodies. In obsessions and compulsions the sense of possession of the thought or act is not impaired, but the patient experiences the obsession as appearing against their will, so that although they have lost control over a voluntary act they still retain personal possession of the act.

In schizophrenia the patient may not only lose the control over their thoughts, actions or feelings, but may also experience them as being foreign or manufactured against their will by some foreign influence. These symptoms are known as ideas or delusions of passivity. The patient may also develop secondary delusions that explain this foreign control as the result of radio waves, X-rays, television, witchcraft, hypnosis, the internet, and so on. This can be described as a delusion of passivity. There is some evidence that delusions of passivity are related to anomalies of the parietal lobe (Maruff et al, 2005), but this association requires further study to clarify the precise anomalies that may underlie these phenomena.

Some individuals with severe anxiety may feel they cannot think clearly or are unable to carry out ordinary volitional activity. They may therefore feel 'as if' they are being controlled by foreign influences. As they have difficulty in thinking and putting their thoughts into words they may give the impression that they know that their thoughts are under foreign control, so it may be difficult to distinguish these 'as if' experiences from true passivity phenomenon, as seen in schizophrenia. This distinction is, however, crucial if misdiagnosis is to be avoided.

Classification of motor disorders

It is difficult to classify motor disorders, because although clear-cut individual motor signs, such as stereotypies, can be treated as if they were neurological symptoms, it is much more difficult to classify more complicated patterns of behaviour. None the less, motor disorders can be broadly grouped into the following:

- disorders of adaptive movements
- disorders of non-adaptive movements
- motor speech disturbances
- disorders of posture
- abnormal complex patterns of behaviour
- movement disorders associated with antipsychotic medication.

Disorders of adaptive movements
Disorders of expressive movement

Expressive movements generally involve the face, arms, hands and the upper trunk. The extent of expressive movement varies with the emotions, but the range of emotional expressions is very different in different cultures and may also differ between individuals in the same culture (for example the use of gesticulation varies across different cultures). Patients with depression tend to have a limited range of expressive movements and may look sad, depressed and anxious. Some patients may try to compensate for their lack of facial expression and reduced mobility in order to mask their depression by smiling; this is colloquially termed 'smiling depression'. Some individuals with depression may weep more frequently than usual, whereas others, especially some of those who are deeply depressed, may state that they feel unable to weep and believe they might feel much better if they could 'have a good cry.'

In severe depression, there may be generalised psychomotor retardation, in which all bodily movements, including gestures, may be diminished or absent. The patient may walk slowly and be bowed down as if carrying a load on their shoulders, and sit with a notable stillness. In agitated or anxious depression, on the other hand, the patient may be restless and apprehensive, sometimes displaying hand-wringing. There is no direct or unvarying relation between the severity of the anxiety and agitation, because some individuals with severe depression who are almost stuperose are in fact extremely anxious.

In schizophrenia, especially with catatonia, expressive movements may also be disordered. The individual with catatonia tends to have a stiff expressive face and the expressive movements of body are similarly scanty. The eyes may appear to be lively, so that the patient appears to be looking at the world through a mask. The flat, full, expressionless face with a greasy appearance (the so-called 'ointment face') may be seen in post-encephalitic parkinsonism, whereas the face tends to be similar but less greasy in Parkinson's disease itself. Excessive grimacing and facial contortions that occur in catatonia are disorders of expression, but are best regarded as stereotypies or the result of parakinesia. In catatonia the lips may be thrust forward in a tubular manner known as 'snout spasm' (*Schnauzkrampf*) and although this is obviously a disorder of expression it is best regarded as a stereotyped posture.

In mania, expressive movements are exaggerated; the patient is unusually cheerful and uses wide expansive gestures. From time to time, transient depression lasting a few seconds may interrupt the manic activity; this is known as emotional lability.

In ecstasy or exaltation the patient has a rapt intense look and is not restless, overactive and interfering. When the ecstasy is extreme the patient is incommunicative and is completely absorbed by the intense experience. In milder ecstatic states the patient may preach or lecture in a high-flown way. Ecstasy is found in certain states of psychosis, schizophrenia, epilepsy and certain personalities with the appropriate religious training.

Disorders of reactive movements

Reactive movements are immediate automatic adjustments to new stimuli, such as occur when an individual flinches in response to a threat or turns towards the source of a novel sound. These movements give rise to a general impression of alertness and adaptation to the environment, so that when they are diminished or lost the patient appears to be stiff and unresponsive in a way that is difficult to describe or designate. Reactive movements are usually affected by obstruction (see below) in catatonia or stupor, so that in addition to the loss of reactive movements there may be obstruction of voluntary movements, which are also carried out in a stiff disjointed manner. Neurological disorders including parkinsonism may lead to a loss of reactive movements. In severe anxiety states reactive movements are prompt and excessive.

Disorders of goal-directed movements

Normal voluntary movements are carried out smoothly without any sense of effort on the part of the individual. They reflect both the personality of the individual and their present mood state. Psychomotor retardation, which occurs in depressive illness, is experienced subjectively as a feeling that all actions have become much more difficult to initiate and carry out. In more severe degrees of psychomotor retardation movements become slow and dragging. The mildest psychomotor retardation can be detected only by careful observation. There is a lack of expression with furrowed eyebrows, the gaze is directed downwards (hence the expression 'to look downcast') and the eyes are unfocused. The individual with agitated depression is easily distracted so that he may have difficulty in initiating a voluntary movement and be unable to carry through a complicated pattern of movements. The execution of individual movements will tend to be prompt once they have been initiated. The individual with mania carries out individual activities swiftly, but the general pattern of behaviour is not consistent.

In some mental illnesses voluntary movements may be performed with difficulty. Psychomotor retardation in depression slows down all psychic and motor acts. In catatonia, blocking or obstruction (also known as *Sperrung*) gives rise to an irregular hindrance to motor activity. We have already encountered hindrance to psychic activity as thought blocking (see above) but here we are considering the effect of blocking on motor acts. Psychomotor retardation has been compared with the uniform slowing down of a vehicle produced by the steady application of a brake, while obstruction has been compared with the effect of putting a rod between the spokes of a moving wheel.

The patient with obstruction may be unable to begin an action at one time and a little later be able to carry it out with no difficulty. Often the patient, when asked to move a part of his body, begins to make a movement and then stops halfway. At times, a voluntary action seems to break through the obstruction and is carried out rather quickly, as if it had to be completed before the obstruction returned. As pointed out above, obstruction may affect habitual and reactive movements, so that the patient does not protect themself when threatened, allow a fly to remain on their face without brushing it off or do not turn towards the speaker when spoken to. Obstruction is common in catatonia and is partly responsible for the stiff ungainly movements that characterise this condition. The muscle tension associated with obstruction may be normal, increased or decreased. The effort needed to overcome obstruction is not related to the muscle tension or the muscles involved, so that it is not dependent on peripheral factors but appears to be a difficulty in carrying out the act itself. This may also manifest as a tendency to react to a request only at the very last moment; for example, the examiner may ask the patient a question and receive no reply, but just as the examiner is turning away the patient answers.

When obstruction is mild, so that spontaneous and reactive movements are only occasionally completely obstructed, the catatonic patient's motor activity appears stiff and awkward. With more severe grades of obstruction akinesia occurs and when the symptom is very marked stupor is present. Severe psychomotor inhibition in psychomotor-retarded depression may also lead to stupor. The different forms of stupor are discussed below (see p. 100).

Individual variation in the execution of goal-directed movements may become so pronounced that the movements are odd and stilted, though still obviously goal-directed. Unusual repeated performances of a goal-directed motor action or the maintenance of an unusual modification of an adaptive posture are known as 'mannerisms'. Examples of this sign are unusual hand movements while shaking hands, when greeting others, and during writing. Other examples may include peculiarities of dress, of hairstyle and writing. The strange use of words, high-flown expressions and movements and postures that are out-of-keeping with the total situation can also be regarded as mannerisms. Some German authors have used the term *bizarreries* as a synonym for mannerisms, while others have defined *bizarreries* as grotesque distorted movements and postures, in which no aim or goal can be see. It must, however, be pointed out that it may be difficult at times to distinguish between mannerisms and stereotypies (see p. 98).

Mannerisms can be found in individuals without mental illness as well as in those with the range of psychiatric disorders and in neurological disorders. In those without psychosis, mannerisms may occur when the person has a need to be noticed, or mannerisms may reflect a lack of control over motor behaviour, possibly associated with a lack of self-confidence (for example a tendency to twirl one's hair around one's finger when speaking in public). This may account for the frequency of mannerisms in adolescence, when teenagers are anxious, insecure and immature and are uncertain how to conduct themselves. In schizophrenia, mannerisms may result from delusional ideas, but may also be regarded as an expression of catatonic motor disorder or a manifestation of 'negativism'.

Mannerisms are not diagnostic of schizophrenia or any other psychiatric illness or disorder. When they occur, their diagnostic significance can only be evaluated if they are regarded as a part of the total clinical picture.

Disorders of non-adaptive movements

Spontaneous movements

Most individuals without mental illness have motor habits that are not goal-directed and that tend to become more frequent during anxiety. Examples of these habits are scratching of the head, stroking, touching or pulling the nose, stroking, scratching or touching the face, putting the hand in front of the mouth, clearing the throat, and so on. These actions have obviously been goal-directed at some time, but have since become spontaneous and not directed towards any goal. Animals prevented from carrying out a normal pattern of behaviour that is usually released by a certain compound stimulus may perform another pattern of movement that is non-adaptive. This is known as displacement activity. The 'normal' motor habits that we are discussing could be regarded as displacement activity as they tend to occur when the individual is frustrated or is uncertain about their choice of behaviour pattern.

Tics are sudden involuntary twitchings of small groups of muscles and are usually reminiscent of expressive movements or defensive reflexes. Commonly the face is affected so that the tic takes the form of blinking, of distortions of the forehead, nose or mouth, but clearing of the throat and twitching of the shoulders may also be tics. Some psychiatrists regard tics as psychogenically determined motor habits, but others believe that the patient has a constitutional predisposition to tics and this is brought to light by emotional tension. In some cases tics have a clear physical basis, when, for example, they occur after encephalitis or indicate the onset of torsion dystonia, Huntington's chorea or Giles de la Tourette syndrome.

Static tremor that occurs in the hands, head and upper trunk when the subject is at rest is another example of a 'normal' spontaneous movement that tends to occur in the very anxious or frightened individual. As not all anxious individuals are markedly tremulous, there is probably an inborn predisposition to tremor. Like any other psychogenic symptom, tremor may occur in the context of conversion disorders. Static tremor may also be familial and tends to worsen as the patient grows older. Despite a fairly marked static tremor of the hands, these individuals are usually able to carry out voluntary movements accurately. Static tremor also occurs in parkinsonism, alcohol dependence syndrome and thyrotoxicosis. Organic tremors vary in intensity from day to day and are made worse by emotional disturbances, so that when a tremor is inconstant and well-marked during a psychological conflict this does not prove that it is solely or fundamentally psychogenic. Intention tremor, which occurs as the goal of the voluntary movement is being reached, is associated with cerebellar disorders and may be seen in multiple sclerosis.

In spasmodic torticollis there is a spasm of the neck muscles, especially the sternomastoid, which pulls the head towards the same side and twists the face in the opposite direction. At first the spasm lasts for a few minutes, but it gradually increases until the neck is permanently twisted. The patient may prevent the movement of the head by holding their chin with their hand.

In chorea, abrupt jerking movements occur that resemble fragments of expressive or reactive movements. In Huntington's chorea the patient may attempt to disguise the choreic movements by turning them into voluntary or habitual ones. For example, the sudden jerking of the arm may be continued into a smoothing down of the hair at the back of the head. If the disease is not too far advanced, this may be mistaken for normal restlessness or overactivity.

In Huntington's chorea, the face, upper trunk and the arms are most affected by the coarse, jerky movements. Snorting and sniffing are often also present. In Sydenham's chorea the movements are less jerky and somewhat slower than in Huntington's chorea. The arms and face are affected and respiration is often irregular because it is made difficult by movements of the spine and the abdominal wall. There is usually widespread hypotonia, sometimes hyporeflexia, and not infrequently a prolongation of the muscular contraction evoked during a tendon reflex (Gordon's phenomenon). In athetosis the spontaneous movements are slow, twisting and writhing, which bring about strange postures of the body, especially of the hands.

There is increasing recognition of, and research interest in, the occurrence of abnormal involuntary movements in individuals with schizophrenia.

While many involuntary movements are associated with antipsychotic medication (Owens, 1999; Gervin & Barnes, 2000) (see below), there is increasing evidence that neurological dysfunction and abnormal involuntary movements are also relatively common in individuals presenting with first episode schizophrenia, prior to the administration of medication. Browne *et al* (2000), for example, found that the majority of neuroleptic-naïve patients with first episode schizophrenia or schizophreniform disorder had significant evidence of neurodysfunction, which was also associated with mixed handedness at time of presentation. While some of the neurological soft signs (for example, motor and cortical signs) appear to be state markers, which may improve as psychopathology improves, other signs ('harder' signs) appear to represent more trait-like, static characteristics, consistent with a neurodevelopmental basis to the illness (Whitty *et al*, 2003). Gervin *et al* (1998) also studied patients with a first episode of schizophrenia or schizophreniform disorder and found that 11.4% had mild orofacial involuntary movements and 7.6% had tardive dyskinesia (repetitive, purposeless movements, usually of the mouth, tongue and facial muscles).

Choreic and athetoid movements are also sometimes encountered in catatonia. Individuals with parakinetic catatonia are in almost constant motion, with grimaces and exaggerated smiles, etc. They may be able to answer simple questions and may be capable of simple routine work. The smile and lack of rigidity may lead to a mistaken diagnosis of hepephrenic schizophrenia in some cases. Some individuals with catatonia may intertwine their fingers or knead and fiddle with the cloth of their clothes. It is difficult to decide whether this sign is a variety of localised parakinesia or a stereotypy.

As pointed out above, a stereotyped movement is a repetitive, non-goal-directed action that is carried out in a uniform way. A stereotypy may be a simple movement or a stereotyped or recurrent utterance. It may be possible to discern the remnants of a goal-directed movement in a stereotypy. In the case of a stereotyped utterance the content may be understandable. Thus an individual with catatonia continuously mumbled the words 'Eesa marider', which appeared to be a corruption of 'He is a married man'. Her illness began when she discovered that her fiancé by whom she was pregnant was a married man. Using Freudian concepts or empathic psychology it may be possible to produce an explanation for the content of a stereotypy, but explaining the content of a symptom does not necessarily explain its form.

Verbal stereotypies or recurring utterances are to be found in expressive aphasia. The neurologist Hughlings Jackson, for example, had a patient with this variety of aphasia following a severe head injury in a brawl, who thereafter could only say 'I want protection'. This is yet another example of the way in which signs and symptoms in catatonia resemble those in neurological disorders.

Abnormal induced movements

Some abnormal induced movements can be regarded as the result of undue compliance on the part of the patient, while others may be interpreted as indicating rejection of the environment. In automatic obedience the patient carries out every instruction regardless of the consequence. To demonstrate this, Emil Kraepelin would ask the patient to put out their tongue and he would prick it with a pin; patients with automatic obedience continued to put their tongue out when asked to, although every time they did so their tongue was pricked. In the past, there has been some confusion about the terms used for this phenomenon; whereas some psychiatrists have used the term 'command automotism' as a synonym for automatic obedience, others have used this term for a syndrome characterised by automatic obedience, waxy flexibility, echolalia and echopraxia. Automatic obedience most commonly occurs in catatonia, although it is also occasionally seen in dementia.

Echopractic patients imitate simple actions that they see, such as hand-clapping, snapping the fingers, and so on. In echolalia the patient echoes a part or the whole of what has been said to them. Words are echoed irrespectively of whether the patient understands them or not, so that the echolalic patient may repeat words and phrases in foreign languages that they do not know. It has been suggested that echo speech in children is a conditional reflex that is suppressed when voluntary speech takes over; echolalia could therefore be seen as the result of disinhibition of a childhood speech pattern. Some individuals, including children, may echo the last words that have been said to them.

Chapman & McGhie (1964) studied echopraxia in individuals with schizophrenia and found that although echopraxia usually took place when the patients were looking at someone else, two patients reported that they echoed the behaviour of a memory image of another person. In some patients echopraxia appeared to be completely automatic, while one patient seemed to decide which person he should imitate.

While stereotypy is a spontaneous abnormal movement, perseveration is an induced movement because it is a senseless repetition of a goal-directed action that has already served its purpose. Thus when a patient is asked to put their tongue out they put it out and then put it in when told to, but continue to put it out and in thereafter. Perseveration is even more obvious when speech is affected because the patient is unable to get beyond a word or phrase, which they go on repeating and may repeat in reply to another question. Logoclonia and palilalia are special forms of perseveration. In the latter, the patient repeats the perseverated word with increasing frequency, while in logoclonia the last syllable of the last word is repeated, for example, the patient might say: 'I am well today-ay-ay-ay-ay.' Palilalia and logoclonia occur in organic brain disorders, in particular in schizophrenia. Perseveration is found in catatonia and organic brain disorders.

Freeman & Gathercole (1966) studied perseveration in schizophrenia, arteriosclerotic dementia and senile dementia. They described three types of perseveration:

- Compulsive repetition, in which the act is repeated until the patient receives another instruction
- Impairment of switching, in which the repetition continues after the patient has been given a new task
- Ideational perseveration, in which the patient repeats words and phrases during their reply to a question.

All three types of perseveration were found in schizophrenia and dementia, but compulsive repetition was more common in individuals with schizophrenia; impairment of switching was more common in individuals with dementia; and ideational perseveration was equally common in both groups.

Forced grasping is most common in catatonia but is also seen in dementia. Forced grasping is demonstrated when the examiner offers his hand to the patient and the patient shakes it (except in cases of negativism). Then the examiner explains that on all future occasions when the examiner offers his hand the patient should not touch it. After this, the examiner talks to the patient for a few minutes and then offers the patient his hand. If forced grasping is present, the patient shakes the examiner's hand. Despite frequent instructions not to touch the examiner's hand the patient continues to do so. The grasp reflex is different; here the patient automatically grasps all objects placed in his hand. Sometimes the reflex has to be produced by drawing an object across the palm of the hand. When unilateral in a fully conscious patient the grasp reflex indicates a frontal lobe lesion on the opposite side, but when bilateral or occurring in clouded consciousness it suggests widespread disorder of the cerebral cortex, which may or may not be reversible. Some patients grope after an object that has stimulated the palm of the hand. If the examiner rapidly touches the palm and steadily withdraws his finger the patient's hand may follow the examiner's finger, rather like a piece of iron following a magnet. This sign has been called the 'magnet reaction' and may occur in catatonia and organic brain disorders.

In cooperation or *Mitmachen*, the body can be put into any position without any resistance on the part of the patient, although they have been instructed to resist all movements. Once the examiner lets go of the body part that has been moved, it returns to the resting position. This disorder is found in catatonia and neurological disease affecting the brain. *Mitgehen* can be regarded as a very extreme form of cooperation, because the patient moves their body in the direction of the slightest pressure on the part of the examiner. For example, the doctor puts his forefinger under the patient's arm and presses gently, whereupon the arm moves upwards in the direction of the pressure. Once the pressure stops the arm returns to its former position. Light pressure on the occiput of the patient, who is standing, leads to bending of the neck, flexing of the trunk and, if the pressure continues, the patient may fall forward. This sign is found in some cases of catatonia when it is usually associated with forced grasping, echolalia and echopraxia. The pressure needed to produce *Mitgehen* is extremely slight, while in cooperation, the movements occur in response to a moderate expenditure of effort on the examiner's part. When examining for *Mitgehen* and cooperation, as in the elicitation of all types of abnormal compliance, the patient must understand that they are expected to resist the examiner's efforts to move them.

Some individuals with catatonia oppose all passive movements with the same degree of force as that which is being applied by the examiner. This is known as *Gegenhalten* or opposition. Often this is not obvious when the passive movements are carried out very gently, and it may only appear when the examiner attempts to produce forceful passive movements.

Negativism can be regarded as an accentuation of opposition. The word negativism is often used to describe hostility, motivated refusal and failure to cooperate; often, these phenomena do not constitute true 'negativism' as they may be goal-directed. Some individuals with severe agitated depression or anxiety and psychosis may be generally apprehensive and try to avoid engagement; it is imprecise to describe this behaviour as negativistic. Negativism is an apparently motiveless resistance to all interference and may or may not be associated with an outspoken defensive attitude. It is found in catatonia, severe learning disability and dementia. Negativism may be passive when all interference is resisted and orders are not carried out, or it may manifest as active or command negativism when the patient does the exact opposite of what they are asked to do, in a reflex way. Some negativistic patients appear to be angry and irritated, while others are blunted and indifferent. Negativism depends to some degree on the environment, so that sometimes there is a special object of the negativistic behaviour. Thus fellow patients may evoke the negativistic reaction much less easily than mental healthcare workers.

Ambitendency can be regarded as a mild variety of negativism or as the result of obstruction. In ambitendency the patient makes a series of tentative movements that do not reach the intended goal when they are expected to carry out a voluntary action. For example, when the examiner puts his hand out to shake hands, the patient moves their right hand towards the examiner's hand, stops, starts moving the hand, stops, and so on, until the hand finally comes to rest without touching the examiner's hand. The patient appears to be in conflict about moving their body and this presence of opposing tendencies to action may be regarded as a form of ambivalence. However, ambitendency is often found in negativistic patients when they are approached carefully and every effort is made to win their confidence. It can then be looked upon as the result of a partial breakdown of the negativistic attitude. If, on the other hand, every effort is not made to win the confidence of the negativistic patient with ambitendency, then the ambitendency may disappear and negativism becomes more obvious. Patients with marked obstruction may make a series of tentative movements before the obstruction prevents all movement. Usually in such a case the body remains for a short period in the position reached when obstruction becomes absolute; in other words, the obstruction is followed by perseveration of posture. This does not occur in ambitendency due to negativism.

Motor speech disturbances in mental disorders

Most of the motor disorders of speech that are found in the psychoses have been mentioned as special examples of other motor signs. At the risk of some repetition, motor speech disorders found in the psychoses will be summarised here.

Attitude to conversation

Patients with negativism tend to turn away from all attempts to speak to them, while other individuals with schizophrenia may experience difficulty maintaining a conversation owing to poor concentration. Other patients with schizophrenia appear to have continuous auditory hallucinations, which make it extremely difficult for them to attend to what is being said. Some patients with catatonia or paraphrenia may whisper continuously and appear to be speaking with hallucinatory voices. Other patients with catatonia turn towards the examiner when he speaks to them and stare at him with an expressionless face, without saying a word; others may turn towards the speaker with a blank face and reply to every question, whether sensible or not. These patients may also talk past the point.

The flow of speech

Some patients with mania or schizophrenia may demonstrate pressure of speech. Individuals with fantastic delusions may become extremely voluble when describing their fantastic experiences and their speech may become very muddled. Some patients with schizophrenia may never stop talking when spoken to and often harangue or lecture the examiner rather than hold a conversation with him.

The quality of speech in catatonia, as in motor aphasia, may be strange and stilted, so that the patient may sound as if they are unfamiliar with the spoken language. Other patients with catatonia may demonstrate unusual intonation, talk in falsetto tone, or have staccato or nasal speech. A few patients with schizophrenia never speak above a whisper or speak with an unusual, strangled voice (*Wurgstimme*). This may be a mannerism or the result of delusions.

Mannerisms and verbal stereotypies

The disorders or stress, inflection and rhythm mentioned in the previous section are mannerisms, but mannerisms of pronunciation also occur. Only a few words may be mispronounced or there may be a distortion of most words, resembling paraphasia. Verbal stereotypies are words or phrases that are repeated. They may be produced spontaneously or be set off by a question. In verbigeration one or several sentences or strings of fragmented words are repeated continuously. For example one of Kraepelin's patients repeated for 3 hours the following sentences: 'Dear Emily, give ma a kiss; we want to get well, a greeting and it would be nothing. We want to be brave and beautiful, follow, follow mother, so that we come home soon. The letter was for me; take care that I get it.'

Sometimes in verbigeration the patient produces strings of incomprehensible jargon in which stereotypies are embedded. Usually the tone of voice is monotonous. Verbigeration is not always spontaneous but may be produced in answer to questions. It is quite different from schizophasia (speech confusion), in which there is gross thought disorder, but the patient speaks in a normal way with changes of intonation and so on.

Perseveration

Verbal perseveration can belong to any of the three types outlined by Freeman & Gathercole (1966) (see above). In some cases there is perseveration of theme rather than the actual words and this can be regarded as impairment of switching. In other cases the set or attitude is perseverated and the patient cannot solve a new problem because they cannot break free from their previous set. Verbal perseveration can occur in schizophrenia and organic states.

Echolalia

As has been pointed out earlier, Stengel (1947) has suggested that echo reactions tend to occur in subjects who wish to communicate, but have permanent or transient receptive and expressive speech disorders. Some patients with catatonia may reply to questions by echoing the content of the question in different words; this is known as echologia.

Disorders of posture

Abnormal postures occur in some individuals in the context of attention-seeking behaviours. Unusual postures may also result from nervous habits in troubled adolescents and individuals with over-anxious personalities. A manneristic posture is an odd stilted posture that is an exaggeration of a normal posture and not rigidly preserved, while a stereotyped one is an abnormal and non-adaptive posture that is rigidly maintained. The exact point at which a postural mannerism becomes a stereotypy may be difficult to decide. Manneristic postures occur in some individuals with schizophrenia, when they may be related to delusional attitudes or catatonia. Although it may be difficult to decide whether some postures are technically manneristic or stereotyped, many stereotyped postures are obvious, as for example when a patient with catatonia sits with their head and body twisted at right angles to a vertical plane passing through both hip joints. Other patients with catatonia lie with their head a few inches off the pillow (a so-called psychological pillow) and maintain this posture for hours. This is a stereotyped posture, which is also seen in dementia.

In perseveration or posture the patient tends to maintain for long periods postures that have arisen fortuitously or which have been imposed by the examiner. The patient allows the examiner to put their body into strange uncomfortable positions and then maintains such postures for at least one minute and usually much longer. Sometimes there is a feeling of plastic resistance as the examiner moves the patient's body, which resembles the bending of a soft wax rod, and when the passive movement stops the final posture is preserved. This is known as waxy flexibility or flexibilitas cerea. In many cases of perseveration of posture there is no resistance to passive movements, but as the examiner releases the body those muscles that fixed the body in the abnormal position can be felt to contract. This is not waxy flexibility and should be called either perseveration of posture or catalepsy.

In some patients catalepsy has to be evoked by putting the patient's arm in a comfortable position, and if this is maintained, the arm is put into a series of unusual positions each of which is more uncomfortable than the previous one, so that finally the patient will preserve very strange postures. If gentle passive movements fail to elicit catalepsy it can sometimes be evoked by moving the arm or limb more firmly into a strange position.

The patient must always be told at first that they are not obliged to leave their body in the position in which it is put by the examiner. If this is not done the patient may believe that they are supposed to maintain the posture as part of the test. One approach is to lift the patient's arm by the wrist and take the pulse; if, when the arm is released, it does not return to the resting position then catalepsy is present, as the individual without catalepsy would naturally realise that they could put their arm down once the examiner has finished feeling the pulse.

Although catalepsy often occurs in the context of mute, stuperose catatonia, it is also found in mild states of akinesia. On occasions it occurs at the same time as obstruction, so that when the obstruction stops, the patient in the middle of an action catalepsy maintains the body in this mid-flight position for some time. Catalepsy usually lasts for more than 1 minute and ends with the body slowly sinking back into the resting position. Catalepsy is often very variable and may disappear for a day or so only to return again. Although waxy flexibility and catalepsy occur in catatonia, they are also seen in conditions such as encephalitis, vascular disorders and neoplasms affecting the mid-brain.

Abnormal complex patterns of behaviour
Non-goal-directed abnormal patterns of behaviour

The two important patterns of behaviour of this type are stupor and excitement, which although dramatically opposed patterns of behaviour, often occur in the same psychiatric disorders.

Stupor

Stupor is a state of more or less complete loss of activity where there is no reaction to external stimuli; it can be regarded as an extreme form of hypokinesia. Psychomotor inhibition and obstruction may produce a general slowing down of activity, and as these disorders become more severe, the patient's condition approaches stupor. Completely stuperose patients are mute, but in sub-stuperose states patients may reply briefly to questions in muttered monosyllables. Stupor may occur in states of shock, dissociative or conversion disorders, depression, psychosis, catatonia and organic brain disease.

Psychogenic stupor may occur in the setting of severe psychological shock, such as those that may occur during bombardment in wartime. The patient is, as it were, 'paralysed with fear' and is unable to retreat from danger. In less severe cases the patient may be virtually mute but not completely motionless and may at times wander about slowly in a small area in a very bewildered way.

Space-occupying lesions affecting the third ventricle, the thalamus and the mid-brain produce a stuperose state in which the eyes are open and the patient appears to be alert, reacts slightly to painful stimuli and is uncooperative. This has been called akinetic mutism, which is a confusing term since these patients have a general lowering of the level of consciousness, failure to register new memories and total amnesia for the episode if they recover.

Stupor may occur in epilepsy when there is continuous epileptic discharge on the electroencephalogram (EEG) or repeated bursts of such discharge. A few patients have recurrent catatonic stupor in which the EEG shows continuous spike and wave discharges. This has been called *'petit mal* status' and is regarded as a special variety of status epilepticus. Patients with Gjessing's periodic catatonia have very slow waves on the EEG during the reaction phase (for example, 2-cycles-per-second).

Although stupor occurs in depression and acute polymorphic psychotic disorder, the most common variety of functional psychosis in which stupor occurs is catatonic schizophrenia. Very occasionally, patients in catatonic stupor have pure akinesia and all muscles are flaccid. Usually the muscle tension is permanently increased or it varies from time to time and is associated with obstruction. At times the muscle tension is so marked that the patient is like a block of wood. The muscle tension in catatonic stupor is usually increased in the muscles of the forehead and the masseters. 'Snout spasm' (*Schnauzkrampf*) is sometimes seen. The sternomastoid muscles are usually contracted, giving rise to the 'psychological pillow.' Opposition or reactive muscle tension may occur. Increased or reactive muscle tension is usually most marked in the anterior neck muscles, the masseters, the muscles around the mouth, and the proximal muscles of the limbs. Tension may be increased permanently or it may disappear and return for varying periods of time. Very rarely all muscles are flaccid with the exception of one group in which tension is markedly increased. The face is usually stiff and devoid of expression, giving rise to a deadpan expression, but often the eyes are lively and contrast with the lack of facial expression. Usually there is no emotional response to affect-laden questions, so that the patient is not disturbed by painful personal questions. As a rule the response to painful stimuli is absent and the patient does not respond to any threat to their existence. Catalepsy may be present. Incontinence of urine is common and incontinence of faeces may occur.

The patient with depressive stupor looks depressed and becomes more depressed when affect-laden topics, such as family affairs, are mentioned. Sometimes the facial expression is more that of anxiety and bewilderment. Catalepsy, obstruction, stereotypies, changes in muscle tone and incontinence of urine and faeces do not occur.

It may be difficult to distinguish between catatonic stupor and depressive stupor. In catatonic stupor, the outstanding features are the deadpan facial expression, changes in muscle tone, catalepsy, stereotypies and incontinence of urine. These are in contrast with the depressive facies, the normal muscle tone, the response to emotional stimuli and the absence of incontinence in depressive stupor. The possibility of a neurological disorder should not be overlooked in a rapidly developing stupor. EEG, computed tomography (CT) of brain and/or lumbar puncture may be required to establish a diagnosis.

Excitement

Although excitement appears to be the opposite of stupor, it often occurs in the same mental illnesses. In some cases it can be understood as being secondary to some other psychological abnormality. Thus in paranoid schizophrenia a sudden increase in the intensity of hallucinatory voices may lead to an excitement. In appreciation-needing personalities, excitements are motivated by a desire for attention or may have the object of imposing a solution of the patient's problems on the environment. In mania the excitement can be understood as a natural consequence of the elated mood. However, some excitements, such as those that occur in catatonia and organic brain disease cannot be understood as arising from some other psychological abnormality.

Psychogenic excitements may be acute reactions or goal-directed reactions. Predisposed subjects may react to moderately stressful situations with senseless violence. This chaotic restlessness may occur in the context of severe stressors (e.g. earthquakes) but may also occur following less severe stresses in certain predisposed individuals (e.g. in some individuals with learning disability). In goal-directed psychogenic reactions excitement may be a part of attention-seeking behaviour; these patients may complain of visual hallucinations but do not show any clear signs of schizophrenia.

Excitement may occur in patients with moderately severe depression, in whom it may take a somewhat mechanical form (for example, the patient may wander about restlessly). In severe agitated depression the patient may rock to and fro, repeatedly lament their situation, and present a picture of abject misery.

In typical manic excitement the patient is cheerful, restless and interfering, with flight of ideas. If the excitement becomes intense, then the patient rushes about the place and may shout incessantly. These patients may rapidly exhaust themselves and develop intercurrent physical illnesses. Usually the mood in hypomania and mania is cheerful, but sometimes the patient is angry and irritable. Such patients may also become violent and threatening when thwarted. Occasionally the mood is one of angry irritation throughout the illness and the patient may become querulous and complaining. In catatonic excitements the face is deadpan and the movements of the body are often stiff and stilted. The violence is usually senseless and purposeless.

In delirium there may be ill-directed overactivity, but occasionally occupational delirium occurs. Many delirious patients are extremely frightened, so that they become more excited when approached by healthcare personnel, whom they think are going to attack them. If the physical condition is not too debilitating, the delirious patient may try to escape his alleged persecution and in doing so kill or harm himself. For example, a delirious patient may jump through a window several stories up in an attempt to escape. Patients with delirium may benefit considerably from reassurance, though it may be necessary to speak loudly and slowly, and to repeat sentences several times.

Pathological drunkenness (also called mania à potu) is a special form of organic excitement, currently classified as pathological intoxication in the *ICD–10 Classification of Mental and Behavioural Disorders* (World Health Organization, 1992). In pathological drunkenness there is an excitement with senseless violence after the patient has drunk a small quantity of alcohol. The episodes may last an hour or so and the patient has amnesia for it. Although it has been termed drunkenness, the patient is not ataxic and does not have the usual signs of drunkenness; intoxication is a preferable term. In some instances, the patient may be murderously aggressive. For example, a British soldier, after drinking a few pints of beer, raked a dance hall with his sub-machine gun, killing 3 people. In another case a man brutally murdered his wife after drinking 3 bottles of beer and in the morning woke up to find himself covered in blood but with no memory for the events leading up to his wife's death.

It is difficult to classify impulsive actions. Here they will be regarded as non-goal-directed complex patterns of behaviour. Most individuals without mental illness have at some time acted on impulse or on the spur of the moment, although some individuals appear more prone to impulsive actions than others. Such individuals may suddenly wander away from their work and homes on impulse, or steal in circumstances in which they are certain to be detected. Impulsive actions, usually of an aggressive kind, are common enough in catatonia. Thus a patient may suddenly strike another, throw a plate or smash a window. It is impossible to find any rational reason for such actions.

Goal-directed abnormal patterns of behaviour

Abnormal patterns of behaviour of this type occur in nearly all psychiatric syndromes, so that only a few such patterns can be discussed here.

Some patients with schizophrenia, especially those with a hebephrenic pattern, behave in a childish, spiteful way to other patients and to staff. They may pull chairs away from other patients who are about to sit down, punch other patients when no one is looking, and so on. Individuals with mania may play practical jokes; for example, one patient would put pieces of coal into the hood of a nurse's coat so that when she pulled her hood over her head she was covered by a shower of coal.

Overall, aggression is not very common in those with mental illness. Surprisingly few individuals with schizophrenia and persecutory ideation actually attack their alleged persecutors. Some people with schizophrenia and gross blunting of affect may become unnecessarily aggressive when thwarted. In first episode psychosis, aggression and violence appear to be particularly associated with drug misuse, involuntary admission status and high psychopathology scores (Foley *et al*, 2005). As pointed out during the discussion of delusions, delusion-like ideas of marital infidelity are more likely to give rise to violent or murderous behaviour than are true delusions of persecution. For example, the jealous husband may beat or even torture his wife in order to extract a 'confession' of infidelity. If an individual with schizophrenia kills someone, they may kill an alleged prosecutor, they may be acting in response to instructions given by hallucinatory voices; or they may be acting in accordance with grandiose religious beliefs. It is worth noting, however, that at a societal level, the proportion of violent crime attributable to schizophrenia is low (Walsh *et al*, 2001) and it is likely that much of the violence associated with schizophrenia is attributable to comorbid substance misuse, which increases risk of violence both in those with mental illness and without mental illness (Steadman *et al*, 1998).

Very rarely, individuals with depression may kill their loved ones before committing suicide themselves. These patients are usually deluded and may believe that they have incurable inherited insanity or some other disease that they have passed on to their children, who are also doomed to suffer. The children are therefore murdered in the mistaken belief that they would be 'better off dead'. This type of murder is known as extended suicide.

The possibility of a relationship between mental illness and suicide bombing associated with terrorism has also been explored by a number of authors in recent years (for discussions see Gordon, 2002; Odelola, 2003; Salib, 2003). Proposed links remain highly controversial, however, and more evidence is needed in order to explore this area further.

Disinhibition resulting from organic brain disease, mania or schizophrenia may give rise to promiscuous behaviour, leading to increased risk of pregnancy and sexually transmitted disease. This may be compounded by downward social drift and reduced attentiveness to physical health as mental illness develops. Increased awareness of the physical health needs of people with mental illness among mental health service providers may help address these issues and minimise long-term risks to patients' health.

There are several other apparently goal-directed abnormal patterns of behaviour that are occasionally seen in the context of mental illness, although it is not always fully clear what the ultimate purpose of the behaviour is. Dissociative fugue, for example, is currently classified as a dissociative (conversion) disorder, characterised by dissociative amnesia, combined with an apparently purposeful journey beyond the patient's usual home or area (World Health Organization, 1992). Although the purpose of the journey may not be fully clear to onlookers, the patient will generally maintain adequate self-care and engage in appropriate simple interactions with others throughout the fugue. As there is amnesia for the period of the fugue, the patient may never be in a position to reveal the purpose of the journey, even after the fugue has ended.

Movement disorders associated with antipsychotic medication

Antipsychotic medication has been associated with a range of movement disorders, including, most notably, extrapyramidal side-effects (Owens, 1999). Many of these movement disorders have already been described and defined in the text above, as some of them (for example, tardive dyskinesia) are associated with mental illness (for example, schizophrenia) prior to the prescription of any medication (Gervin et al, 1998).

In summary, movement disorders associated with antipsychotic medication include acute akathisia (restlessness or inability to keep still), chronic akathisia, acute dystonia (involuntary sustained muscle contraction or spasm), tardive dystonia, and acute and tardive dyskinesia (repetitive, purposeless movements, usually of the mouth, tongue and facial muscles) (Gervin & Barnes, 2000). In addition to the externally observable signs associated with these extrapyramidal side-effects, it is important also to elicit the psychological or subjective components of these effects (Owens, 2000). Akathisia, in particular, may be associated with subjective restlessness, tension and general unease. Tardive dyskinesia may lead to significant additional stigmatisation and social disability.

Systematic examination for these movement disorders, both prior to medication and during treatment, is critical for the prevention, diagnosis and management of ongoing movement disorder. Examination may involve careful clinical examination and the use of appropriately validated rating scales (Owens, 1999; Gervin & Barnes, 2000). Management may involve reducing antipsychotic dose, changing to another medication, or prescribing additional medication (for example, anticholinergic agents), depending on the side-effects present and the individual clinical circumstances (Taylor et al, 2003).

References

Browne, S., Clarke, M., Gervin, M., *et al* (2000) Determinants of neurological dysfunction in first episode schizophrenia. *Psychological Medicine*, **30**, 1433–1441.

Chapman, J. & McGhie, A. (1964) Echopraxia in schizophrenia. *British Journal of Psychiatry*, **110**, 365–374.

Foley, S. R., Kelly, B. D., Clarke, M., *et al* (2005) Incidence and clinical correlates of aggression and violence at presentation in patients with first episode psychosis. *Schizophrenia Research*, **72**, 161–168.

Freeman, T. & Gathercole, C. E. (1966) Perseveration – the clinical symptoms in chronic schizophrenia and organic dementia. *British Journal of Psychiatry*, **112**, 27–32.

Gervin, M. & Barnes, T. R. E. (2000) Assessment of drug-related movement disorders in schizophrenia. *Advances in Psychiatric Treatment*, **6**, 332–341.

Gervin, M., Browne, S., Lane, A., *et al* (1998) Spontaneous abnormal involuntary movements in first-episode schizophrenia and schizophreniform disorder: baseline rate in a group of patients from an Irish catchment area. *American Journal of Psychiatry*, **155**, 1202–1206.

Gordon, H. (2002) The 'suicide' bomber: is it a psychiatric phenomenon? *Psychiatric Bulletin*, **26**, 285–287.

Maruff, P., Wood, S. J., Velakoulis, D., *et al* (2005) Reduced volume of parietal and frontal association areas in patients with schizophrenia characterized by passivity delusions. *Psychological Medicine*, **35**, 783–789.

Odelola, D. (2003) Suicide bombers and institutional racism. *Psychiatric Bulletin*, **27**, 358.

Owens, D. G. C. (1999) *A Guide to the Extrapyramidal Side-Effects of Antipsychotic Drugs*. Cambridge: Cambridge University Press.

Owens, D. G. C. (2000) Commentary on: assessment of drug-related movement disorders in schizophrenia. *Advances in Psychiatric Treatment*, **6**, 341–343.

Salib, E. (2003) Suicide terrorism: a case of folie à plusiers? *British Journal of Psychiatry*, **182**, 475–476.

Steadman, H. J., Mulvey, E. P., Monahan, J., *et al* (1998) Violence by people discharged from acute psychiatric inpatient facilities and by others in the same neighborhoods. *Archives of General Psychiatry*, **55**, 393–401.

Stengel, E. (1947) A clinical and psychological study of echo reactions. *Journal of Mental Science*, **93**, 598–612.

Taylor, D., Paton, C. & Kerwin, R. (2003) *The South London and Maudsley NHS Trust: 2003 Prescribing Guidelines*. London: Martin Dunitz.

Walsh, E., Buchannan, A. & Fahy, T. (2001) Violence and schizophrenia: examining the evidence. *British Journal of Psychiatry*, **180**, 490–495.

Whitty, P., Clarke, M., Browne, S., *et al* (2003) Prospective evaluation of neurological soft signs in first-episode schizophrenia in relation to psychopathology: state versus trait phenomena. *Psychological Medicine*, **33**, 1479–1484.

World Health Organization (1992) *The ICD–10 Classification of Mental and Behavioural Disorders: Clinical descriptions and diagnostic guidelines* (10th edn). Geneva: WHO.

CHAPTER 9

Personality disorders

Although personality disorder has no specific psychopathology, the problems associated with its distinction from Axis I disorders justifies its inclusion. True to the Germanic tradition of Schneider, who believed there was overlap between personality disorder and the neuroses, the *ICD−10 Classification of Mental and Behavioural Disorders* (ICD−10; World Health Organization, 1992) does not distinguish them either and classifies them on a single axis, whereas the *Diagnostic and Statistical Manual of Mental Disorders* (DSM−IV; American Psychiatric Association, 1994) classifies personality disorder on a separate axis from mental state disorders.

The history of personality disorder is one of the oldest in psychiatry dating back to Hippocrates, who believed that the balance between the four humours represented the different elements of personality, being identified as yellow bile from the liver, black bile from the spleen, blood and phlegm. These represented choleric (bad-tempered), melancholic (gloomy), sanguine (optimistic/confident) and phlegmatic (placid/apathetic) traits respectively.

The person who contributed most to our modern understanding of personality is undoubtedly Schneider, although his work *Psychopathic Personalities for Modern Classificatory Schemes*, first published in 1923, was not translated into English until 1950. He defined those with personality disorder as 'those who suffer or make society suffer on account of their abnormality', a view that is found in both of the contemporary classifications. He used the term 'psychopathic' in a broad sense to describe the totality of personality disorders, although this term has had a more restricted use in recent decades.

Definition

Personality can be defined as the totality of the person's emotional and behavioural traits that characterise their day-to-day living. Personality disorders are deeply ingrained, maladaptive patterns of behaviour, generally recognisable by adolescence and continuing throughout adult life.

Dimensions and categories

The modern understanding of personality is derived from trait psychology and it places traits on a continuum from absent to severe. Only those traits that reach a threshold for severity (impinging on self or others negatively) are regarded as pathological. In order to diagnose a specific personality disorder it is necessary to have a cluster of traits that are at or above this threshold. However, since most of the categories of personality disorder classified in ICD–10 and DSM–IV have not been validated and overlap with each other, there is debate about whether this categorical approach is the best way to conceptualise personality. Although the trait approach is currently in the ascendancy, others argue for a dimensional approach where every trait is measured on a continuum and rather than assuming discrete categories as if each was an ontological entity, each person's personality is described across a range of dimensions and the distinction between personality disorder and its absence disappears.

Most studies have identified four or five dimensions that cover the broad areas of sociability, neuroticism, obsessionality and dissocial behaviour, although these have been accorded different names by the various researchers. For example, Tyrer & Alexander (1979) identified schizoid, passive–dependent, anankastic and sociopathic dimensions; Livesley *et al* (1998) described emotional dysregulation, dissocial, inhibitedness and compulsivity dimensions; and Mulder & Joyce (1997) described the four A's, 'antisocial, asocial, asthenic and anankastic'. Costa & McCrea (1992a) have developed a five-factor model of personality, with dimensions called neuroticism, extraversion, openness to experience, agreeableness and conscientiousness. A detailed review of the dimensional approach is provided by Tyrer (2005) and by Widiger & Simonsen (2005).

Notwithstanding the aspirations to replace categories with dimensions, this change is unlikely to happen soon, largely due to the long tradition attaching to the current categorical approach and because categories facilitate communication between mental health professionals in a way that dimensions may never achieve.

Assessing personality

Clinical assessment

Since this is the most common method by which personality is assessed in practice, it is important to have a proper understanding of its methods and pitfalls. It is imperative that the assessment of personality takes place when the person has recovered from an episode of illness, since Axis I mental state disorder can contaminate the person's view of his or her personality. For example, the person with depression may describe themselves as always having few friends or as lacking in any talent or ability. In addition their demeanor may also give the impression of personality disorder, so that the downcast eyes of the person with depression or the irritability present in hypomania may create an impression of shyness or of irascibility.

If personality is to be assessed while the person is still ill, then information must be obtained from those who know the person well; this may be relatives, friends or the family doctor. However, it is essential to emphasise that it is traits that have been present throughout adult life that are of interest and not just traits observed during the most recent episode of illness. This distinction can be difficult for some to make, especially when the duration of the current episode of illness has been lengthy, chronic or treatment-resistant. Inevitably this makes personality assessment problematic in those with residual schizophrenia.

Since nobody is perfect, it is inevitable that abnormal traits will be present to some extent in every person. Some novices find it difficult to make the distinction between these and personality disorder. The distinction resides in the impact that the traits have on the person and on others. Impacting on others in a negative manner is a requirement in both DSM–IV and ICD–10, although DSM–IV also allows for the lesser criterion of personal distress. Thus using DSM–IV the prevalence of personality disorder is likely to be higher than using ICD–10, although the detailed specification for each disorder in DSM is likely to counterbalance this. Whichever classification is used, it is essential to evaluate the impact of the traits on the person and on others also. If there is no impact, or if the functional impairment is low, then a diagnosis of personality disorder should not be made.

Older instruments

The Minnesota Multiphasic Personality Inventory (MMPI; Hathaway & McKinley, 1940) is still commonly used by psychologists to obtain a personality profile. It does not make categorical diagnoses and was developed to differentiate between the categories of abnormal personality among in-patients, but it has also been extensively studied in the healthy population. The subject is presented with 550 statements and asked to respond to each with 'true', 'false' or 'cannot say'. Unfortunately the scales have been labelled using the standard nosology of psychiatry (for example, paranoia, schizophrenia, psychopathy, etc.), therefore interpretation by an experienced psychologist is required.

The Eysenck Personality Inventory (EPI; Eysenck & Eysenck, 1964) is probably still the best-known instrument and its simplicity of use makes it appealing. It consists of 108 questions relating to the three dimensions of neuroticism, extroversion and psychoticism, as well as a lie scale. Although widely used in studies of physical and psychiatric disorders, it suffers from the problem that current psychiatric disorder will markedly influence the neuroticism (N) scale.

Screening instruments

These screen for the possibility of personality disorder and are therefore quick to administer. The Iowa Personality Disorder Screen (IPDS; Langbehn *et al*, 1999) consists of 11 screening items for the DSM−IV categories and takes 5−10 minutes to administer. It shows a high sensitivity and specificity. The Standardised Assessment of Personality (SAP; Mann *et al*, 1981) is an informant scale that can be used for screening although it is more often used as a full personality assessment tool. The Standardised Assessment of Personality Abbreviated Scale (SAPAS; Moran *et al*, 2003) consists of 8 dichotomously rated items from SAP (Mann *et al*, 1981) completed by the subject. It shows good sensitivity and specificity and may prove feasible for use in everyday clinical practice. The Personality Assessment Schedule (PAS; Tyrer & Alexander, 1979) has a screening version (PAS−Q), which takes a few minutes to administer to the subject, but it can be used only by an interviewer already trained in the use of PAS.

Structured assessment

Questionnaires

Although questionnaires, such as the Millon Clinical Multiaxial Inventory (MCMI; Millon, 1982) and the Personality Disorder Questionnaire (PDQ; Hyler *et al*, 1990) are convenient to use, they have the serious disadvantage of generating high false-positive rates due to overdiagnosis. The MCMI is a self-administered questionnaire of 175 items. It takes 25 minutes to complete and analysis is by computer. It provides an individual profile, an interpretive report, and a categorical assessment of personality limited to borderline, schizotypal and paranoid types. The most popular personality questionnaire the Neuroticism, Extraversion, Openness Personality Inventory (NEO−PR; Costa & McCrae, 1992*b*) consists of 250 self-rating items measured on a 5-point Likert scale. The ease of use of questionnaires, taking no more than minutes to self-rate by the subject, is also their disadvantage, since they are incapable of distinguishing mental state features from personality traits.

Interviews

Structured interviews such as the PAS (Tyrer & Alexander, 1979) and the Diagnostic Interview for DSM−IV Personality Disorders (DIPD−IV; Zanarini *et al*, 1994) achieve good reliability, but are lengthy instruments and require training in their use. Other distinctions lie in their use of informants or subjects or both, an important consideration since there is evidence to suggest that reliability is higher with informants than with subjects alone (Modestin & Puhan, 2000).

The PAS generates diagnoses both for ICD−10 and DSM−IV. It requires either the subject or the informant or both to provide information on 24 traits of personality, and emphasis throughout is placed on the patient's premorbid traits. It takes 30−40 minutes to administer.

The Structured Interview for DSM−III Personality Disorders (SID−P; Pfohl *et al*, 1983) is a comprehensive semi-structured interview with 60 items. Data are gathered from the subject and an informant to generate the diagnosis.

The Personality Disorder Examination (Loranger *et al*, 1985) is a lengthy structured interview with 359 items, some traits and some behavioural measures, which also generates both DSM–IV and ICD–10 diagnoses. It takes around 3 hours to complete and its size precludes its use except in research settings. The Structured Clinical Interview for DSM–II (SCID–II) was developed by Spitzer *et al* (1987) to focus exclusively on Axis II diagnosis and has been adapted to make DSM–IV diagnoses. The interview commences by administering the Personality Disorder Questionnaire (PDQ) (Hyler *et al*, 1990) and the subject is requested to make a series of dichotomous yes/no choices. The SCID–II interview then focuses on questions to which a positive response has already been given, covering all the traits in the DSM–IV personality disorder section, but the interviewer makes the diagnosis.

Categorical classification

Although the use of categories continues in clinical practice, there is overlap between the individual categories; one study found that 34 subjects received a total of 92 Axis II diagnoses (Sara *et al*, 1996). In addition there is poor inter-rater reliability with the exception of the antisocial category (Zimmerman, 1994).

Table 9.1   DSM–IV and ICD–10 personality disorders

DSM–IV	ICD–10	Main features
Cluster A		
Paranoid	Paranoid	Suspicious, feelings of perception
Schzoid	Schizoid	Cold, detached, isolated
Schizotypal	(1)	Isolated, eccentric ideas
Cluster B		
Antisocial	Dissocial	Behaviour disorder, callous, antisocial
	Emotionally unstable personality	acts
Borderline	a. impulsive	Instability of mood, behaviour, unstable
(2)	b. borderline	relationships
Histrionic	Histrionic	Shallow, dramatic, egocentric
Narcissistic	(3)	Self-centred, grandiosity, entitlement
Cluster C		
Avoidance	Anxious	Hypersensitive, timid, self-conscious
Dependent	Dependent	Submissive, helplessness
Obsessive–compulsive	Anakastic	Doubt, caution, obsessional

(1) Schizotypal disorder is classified in the section on schizophrenia
(2) Impulsive personality disorder is in ICD–10 but not DSM–IV, which instead includes intermittent explosive disorder as an impulse control disorder separate from personality disorder
(3) Narcissistic personality disorder is not included in ICD–10

The categories listed in DSM–IV and ICD–10 are shown in Table 9.1 and some have different names in each.

DSM–IV recognises three clusters of personality disorder, although ICD–10 does not organise the categories into groups. Nevertheless, this clustering does provide a useful way of grouping disorders, particularly for research purposes:

1.   Cluster A or the eccentric group incorporates the paranoid, schizoid and schizotypal categories
2.   Cluster B or the dramatic group includes the histrionic, borderline, narcissistic and antisocial categories
3.   Cluster C or the fearful group includes the obsessive–compulsive, avoidant and dependent groups.

Clinical descriptions of categories

Paranoid personality disorder

These people are touchy and take umbrage easily. They believe that people have malevolent intentions towards then and they fail to trust those whom they should, such as parents or spouses. They have great difficulty accepting reassurance that they are not the victim of plots and often alienate their friends, living lives of isolation, further compromising their reality testing. They may also become pathologically jealous and overly suspicious of the intentions of others towards their spouses and friends. They sometimes resort to litigation for relatively minor reasons. Along with overvalued ideas of suspicion they may also display grandiosity and they can decompensate into psychotic states when delusions replace the overvalued ideas. Insight is usually lacking since others are perceived as to blame for the problems and such people rarely present for treatment of the primary disorder except perhaps with pathological jealousy when the spouse initiates referral. In practice, it is often difficult to separate paranoid personality disorder from the equivalent psychotic state (persistent delusional disorder). A complication that can arise in old age is the Diogenes syndrome (see Appendix I), in which the person chooses to live in squalor; many such people have a history suggestive of paranoid personality disorder.

Schizoid personality disorder

Although first described by Bleuler (1922), who believed it had an association with schizophrenia, recent studies have shown this to be incorrect and that instead the presumed association represents the prodromal phase of the illness itself.

Schizoid personality disorder is characterised by aloofness, detachment and emotional coldness. There is little interest in human relationships and the person with this disorder is often described as introspective with a greater enthusiasm for philosophy or art than for people. Not surprisingly they do not form long-term relationships and rarely present for treatment

111

unless some Axis I disorder develops. The differential diagnosis is from anxious (avoidant personality) disorder, but in the latter there is a strong desire to have relationships but an inability to do so owing to shyness and poor social skills. The early phase of schizophrenia with social withdrawal may resemble schizoid personality disorder and only time will clarify the diagnosis as psychotic symptoms emerge. The feeling of detachment that characterises depersonalisation may be confused with the emotional detachment of the person with schizoid personality disorder. However, the latter describes their detachment as distressing and it has the subjective quality of being cut-off or 'outside' oneself, whereas no such distress attaches to schizoid personality disorder. Schizoid personality disorder must also be distinguished from Asperger syndrome. As well as speech abnormalities, Asperger syndrome is characterised by social gaucheness in the realm of social interactions, in which the nuances of social behaviour governing posture, gesture, proxemics, eye contact, and personal empathy are lacking. Those with Asperger syndrome may get teased at school and so withdraw from social contact and appear to have schizoid personality disorder, not because of any desire to do so, but as a result of an awareness that they are different from others.

Schizotypal personality disorder (DSM–IV only)

In view of the association with schizophrenia, this disorder is classified with schizophrenia rather than with personality disorders in ICD–10. Like people with schizoid personalities, those with schizotypal personalities are aloof and isolated but they do have a feeling of involvement in the world and have the capacity to form relationships to some extent. At other times they feel detached from the world, describe depersonalisation and isolate themselves. During these periods they communicate in an odd manner and affect is inappropriate. There may be ideas of reference, odd beliefs not amounting to delusions, magical thinking and suspiciousness. The distinction from prodromal schizophrenia is difficult to make.

Histrionic personality disorder

Histrionic and hysterical personality disorders are often used interchangeably. This personality disorder is characterised by seductive and overdramatic behaviour. Others are essential to maintaining the person's self-esteem. In contrast to the dependent personality, histrionic individuals take the initiative in the quest for nurture, and this leads to seductive and overdramatic behaviour.

This category has always been controversial and although described in great detail it is seldom diagnosed. One of the difficulties is that it carries overtones of sexism as it may be seen as a caricature of femininity (Chodoff & Lyons, 1958) and is more frequently diagnosed in women than men, often without due regard to the criteria necessary for making the diagnosis (Thompson & Goldberg, 1987).

The core features are self-dramatisation, lability of mood, sexual provocativeness, egocentricity and excessive demand for praise and approval. Initially there is an appearance of openness and social skill: however, this is also mixed with shallow, flirtatious and manipulative behaviour. Hyperbolic speech and melodramatic descriptions are noticeable and anything but the most superficial of introspection is lacking. Those with histrionic personality disorder are prone to anxiety related to separation and although it was once thought that it was linked to conversion and dissociative disorders, recent research shows that this is incorrect (Chodoff & Lyons, 1958). Somatisation is often associated with this personality disorder in a condition known as Briquet's syndrome. Short-lived histrionic features are sometimes observed in those with depressive illness and with hypomania and this should not be called personality disorder. There are those who believe that this diagnosis should be relegated to the group of personality disorders that requires further study (Dowson & Grounds, 1995) owing to the paucity of recent research.

Emotionally unstable personality disorder

ICD–10 subsumes two personality disorder categories under this rubric. These are impulsive personality disorder and borderline personality disorder. However, DSM–IV classifies borderline personality disorder on its own, and in a group termed 'habit disorders' describes a condition resembling impulsive personality called intermittent explosive disorder.

Impulsive personality disorder

This is characterised by poor impulse control with explosive outbursts. The person has little consideration of the consequences and an inability to plan ahead. Its nearest equivalent in DSM–IV, intermittent explosive disorder, is characterised by outbursts that are disproportionate to any precipitating stressor, sometimes a surge of energy prior to the outbursts followed by lowering of mood and remorse. Although it is diagnosed more frequently in men, some women describe similar episodes premenstrually. In view of the favourable response to selective serotonin reuptake inhibitors (SSRIs) and mood stabilisers there have been inevitable suggestions of a link to bipolar disorder.

Borderline personality disorder

Standing on the border between neurosis and psychosis, this disorder is characterised by extraordinary instability of behaviour, affect, mood and self-image. There is impulsivity of behaviour with repeated self-harm, often cutting, being used to express anger, seek attention or numb the emotional pain. Feelings of boredom and emptiness are often described and there is intolerance of being alone, often resulting in a frantic search for company and promiscuous behaviour. Disorders of body-image and doubts about gender identity are common. Since fear of abandonment and splitting (seeing people as all bad or all good) are central to the borderline view of the world, relationships are fraught. There is a tendency to intense and idealised dependence, only to later spurn and direct aggression to the loved one. Because of shifting allegiances these patients may cause disharmony between individuals or groups, for example, between nurses and doctors on the ward. Mood swings and crises are common and the person may vacillate between anger, low mood and having no feelings at all in short succession. A history of abuse, sexual or physical, is common and believed to be of aetiological significance. Short-lived psychotic episodes, known as micropsychotic episodes, may occur but resolve rapidly and at times there may be doubts about the presence of psychotic symptoms if the symptoms are vague. Projective identification, i.e. the projection of intolerable aspects of self onto another, who is then induced to act in a manner similar to the projector, is common and therapists should be aware of this so that they do not become part of the patient's distorted world. Because of the intensity of emotions and the impulsive behaviour patients do not reach their academic or employment potential. It has a number of trenchant critics, including Tyrer (2002), who comments that borderline personality disorder is 'a controversial diagnosis of such overwhelming comorbidity that it embraces the whole of psychiatry'.

Dissocial personality disorder

The core features of this personality disorder are callousness and lack of empathy. The person is unable to comprehend how their cruel or callous behaviour might affect others, and although there may be a superficial ,recognition of the mores of society their apologies are superficial, remorse is absent and there is little learning from experience or from punishment; 'Do unto others as you would have them do unto you' has little meaning for the dissocial person.

As the boredom threshold is low, these individuals resort to thrill-seeking behaviours such as substance misuse, gambling and promiscuity. Some are superficially charming and form relationships, though these are often short-lived, and there may be a history of serial marriages or cohabitations, ending due to infidelity or violence. Others are more obviously cold and hard and get pleasure from hurting those close to them. Although the diagnosis is more commonly made in men, women are not precluded. They may present with a history of neglecting or abandoning their children or abusing their spouse or partner. Since those with dissocial personality disorder lie, their history may be unreliable. They frequently have a history, beginning in childhood, of conduct disorder, attention-deficit hyperactivity disorder, truancy, cruelty to animals, fights and substance misuse. Suicide threats and behaviour are common, and although mood may be low, this is generally in response to thwarted plans and resolves rapidly. The dissocial person uses the defence mechanisms of projection, in which others are blamed for causing the behaviour, and rationalisation, claiming justification. However, their veneer of civility assists them in employment and relationships, but as it drops, they alienate others, leading to major social dysfunction.

Dissocial personality disorder must be distinguished from the secondary effects of alcohol and drug misuse that lead to criminal behaviour but which is absent in the absence of substance misuse. This is particularly difficult when the substance misuse began in adolescence and it may be impossible to distinguish which is the primary psychopathology.

Both men and women may at times be violent, but it must be emphasised that most violent people do not have dissocial personality disorder, and therefore criminality is not synonymous with this diagnosis. During a manic episode there may be risk-taking behaviour and aggression but the history should clarify the diagnosis. Some brain lesions may lead to behaviour and personality change resembling that seen in the dissocial person, but a clear history of trauma will clarify the diagnosis. Some adolescents from deprived backgrounds may display antisocial characteristics into early adulthood but with maturation become well-adjusted and functional people. It would be inappropriate to apply this label to a young person in these circumstances and the diagnosis should only be made after detailed history-taking, especially from others and when the features have been present into adult life. Among women the differentiation from borderline personality disorder may also be problematic, but the latter does not have the core of callousness or remorselessness.

Anankastic (obsessive–compulsive) personality disorder

Referred to as the obsessive–compulsive category in DSM–IV, this category of personality disorder was first described by Freud in 1908. There is, if anything, a likelihood that anankastic personality disorder will be overdiagnosed since the traits, being generally regarded as virtues, are often described in clinical settings. There is a danger that inexperienced doctors will label a patient who describes liking a routine, being punctual, having high standards and being neat as meeting the criteria for this disorder, without any requirement for distress or a negative impact on others. It is crucial therefore not to set the threshold for diagnosis too low.

The main features include punctuality, neatness, difficulty with uncertainty, yet a great need to be in control. Chance has to be reduced to a minimum, and any unplanned situation avoided. Such individuals like routine and may have a timetable for each day, which is not permitted to vary from week to week. They may be rigid in their views, lack spontaneity and in extreme cases insist on others adhering to their views and their timetables, leading to disagreements. Thus going out with friends on the spur of the moment is difficult and everything, such as holidays, is planned with care and precision. They present as neat, stiff and formal, though they are rarely referred for this reason alone since these traits, in a milder form, may be valued by society and so the diagnosis is most commonly made during an assessment of an Axis I disorder.

115

Dependent personality disorder

This is characterised by excessive emotional reliance on other people and as lacking in confidence. Individuals with this disorder need assistance in making simple decisions and present as lacking in ambition and as compliant with the wishes of others. They may describe being taken advantage of in social and employment situations and may sometimes be the victims of bullying. Appearing to be self-effacing and humble, they often underplay their abilities. Their demeanour is passive and this may show itself in posture, tone of voice, etc. Feelings of loneliness are often described since they may have difficulty making long-term relationships owing to the emotional demands they place on others. Alternatively they become involved with very assertive partners and have seemingly happy relationships. Distress is easily engendered by day-to-day problems of living owing to their limited resources for problem solving and decision-making. A pattern similar to dependent personality disorder may develop following bereavement or during a depressive episode but this resolves over time and should not be equated with personality disorder.

Anxious (avoidant) personality disorder

Those with anxious personality disorder feel their need for friendship very acutely yet lack the social skills necessary to even begin to form these relationships. They are shy, tense and easily embarrassed. As a result they are isolated and lonely yet have an overwhelming need to be accepted, while also being unsure of their self-worth. The more artistically able among them tend to compensate by engaging in solitary intellectual pursuits such as music, art, literature and poetry, from which they derive some comfort. They may be able to enter long-term relationships with those who can offer uncritical acceptance.

The distinction from social anxiety can be difficult to make and some argue that anxious personality disorder is a mild form of social anxiety disorder (Fahlen, 1995). However, there are differences; anxious personality disorder is more generalised, with fear extending to multiple areas of social encounters, whereas social anxiety disorder is more limited to one of a few areas, for example speaking in public or eating in front of others. In addition pervasive low self-esteem and an excessive desire for acceptance are not part of the pattern of social anxiety disorder. Nevertheless, in spite of these distinctions there is considerable overlap (Fahlen, 1995) and it can be very difficult clinically to distinguish one from the other. It must also be distinguished from schizoid personality disorder; people with the latter disorder have no interest in personal relationships, while those with anxious personality disorder have an intense desire to make friends. Those experiencing a depressive illness may also describe problems in dealing with people, leading to social withdrawal as well as specific problems answering the telephone, the door, etc., although the recency of onset will clarify the diagnosis.

Other categories

Narcissistic personality disorder

This category is not included in ICD−10 and the diagnosis is rarely made outside the USA. Its continuing inclusion in DSM−IV in the Cluster B group, demonstrates the continuing influence of Freudian psychoanalysis in America. People with this disorder have a grandiose sense of self-importance. They may be preoccupied by fantasies of success, power and brilliance and believe it is their right to receive special treatment. Their self-esteem is based on a grandiose assumption of personal worth. However, their feelings of superiority are fragile, and there may be an exhibitionistic need for constant attention and admiration from others. Feelings of envy are directed at those whom they perceive as being more successful. They exaggerate their personal worth and may show interpersonal exploitativeness and lack empathy, entering relationships only if they believe it will profit them. In romantic relationships, the other partner is often treated as little more than an object to bolster their self-esteem. They are often described as arrogant. A high degree of egocentricity occurs in many of the other personality disorders, and so this trait is not in itself diagnostic. In antisocial personality disorder it is associated with a more malevolent feeling towards others, while those with narcissistic personalities are well-disposed, believing that other people admire them. They are less impulsive and emotional than those with borderline disorder, less dramatic than patients with histrionic personality disorder, and are more cohesive and successful than those with dependent personality disorder. However, in practice any of the above disorders may coexist with narcissistic personality disorder.

Passive aggressive personality disorder

Passive aggressive personality disorder is not included in ICD−10, and in DSM−IV it appears only in the appendix 'Criteria sets and axes provided for further study', indicating doubt concerning the validity of the disorder. The name is based on the assumption that people with this disorder are covertly expressing aggression. It is characterised by a pervasive pattern of passive resistance in both the domestic and work situation and manifests itself indirectly by procrastination, stubbornness, intentional inefficiency and forgetfulness. Those with this disorder become sulky or irritable when asked to do something they do not wish to do. The clinical picture shows some resemblance to oppositional defiant disorder of childhood and adolescence, which is a much more severe condition.

Depressive personality disorder

This category is not included in ICD−10 and in DSM−IV is only included in the section entitled 'Criteria sets and axes provided for further study'. It refers to a lifelong depressive temperament with a pervasive pattern of depressive cognitions and behaviour, pessimism and low self-esteem.

These individuals may also be judgemental and negative about others, and are viewed as unduly pessimistic and humourless. The distinction from dysthymia is difficult to make and depressive personality disorder and dysthymia are frequently comorbid. Although it is not included in DSM−IV, there is some support for the inclusion of depressive personality disorder in DSM−V as a specific category on the basis of the stability of the depressive traits over time (Phillips *et al*, 1998).

Mixed personality disorders (ICD−10) and personality disorder not otherwise specified (DSM−IV): only a minority of patients can be easily placed in one of the specific diagnostic categories outlined in the preceeding sections. The majority of patients with a personality disorder have traits that fulfil criteria for a mixture of two or three personality disorders and in these cases DSM−IV recommends that two or three separate personality disorders should be recorded, while ICD−10 recommends a diagnosis of 'mixed personality disorder'.

Enduring personality changes after a catastrophic experience

Although uncommon, it is now recognised that a person's character may change as a consequence of stressful events, particularly if the stress was extreme. ICD−10 describes a category in which the onset of the changed personality can be traced to a particular event or illness, such as a catastrophic experience or an episode of severe psychiatric illness even though it is now resolved. The clinical picture is usually one of social withdrawal, coupled with a somewhat hostile or mistrustful attitude to the world. Subjects may complain of feelings of hopelessness, estrangement, and a chronic feeling of being on edge, as if constantly threatened. The diagnosis should only be made if the personality changes have lasted more than 2 years. The disorder is difficult to differentiate from chronic post-traumatic stress disorder and the latter may precede it. When it follows an episode of psychiatric illness the clinical picture is mainly one of dependency, a demanding attitude to others, reduced interests and passivity, with persistent claims of being ill-associated with illness behaviour, dysphoria, and impaired occupational and social function. In making this diagnosis there should be no evidence of premorbid personality disorder. Further study is required to confirm the validity of this category of personality disorder since it was first introduced in ICD−10 in 1992.

There is no precise equivalent in DSM−IV, but it does include a section on 'personality change due to a medical condition'. Personality changes can also occur due to organic brain disease.

References

American Psychiatric Association (1994) *Diagnostic and Statistical Manual of Mental Disorders* (4th edn) (DSM−IV). Washington DC: APA.

Bleuler, E. (1922) [Die probleme der schizoidie und der syntonie.] *Zeitschrift für die Gesamte Neurologie und Psychiatrie*, **78**, 373−388.

Chodoff, P. & Lyons, H. (1958) Hysteria, the hysterical personality and 'hysterical' conversion. *American Journal of Psychiatry*, **114**, 734–740.

Costa, P. T. & McCrea, R. R. (1992*a*). The five-factor model of personality and its relevance to personality disorders. *Journal of Personality Disorder*, **6**, 343–359.

Costa, P. T. Jr & McCrae, R. R. (1992*b*) *Revised NEO Personality Inventory (NEO-PI-R) and NEO Five-Factor Inventory (FFI) Manual*. Odessa, FL: Psychological Assessment Resources.

Dowson, J. H. & Grounds, A. T. (1995) *Personality Disorders: Recognition and Clinical Management*. Cambridge: Cambridge University Press.

Eysenck, H. & Eysenck, S. B. G. (1964) *Manual of the Eysenck Personality Inventory (EPQ)*. London: University of London Press.

Fahlen, T. (1995) Personality traits in social phobia. Comparison with healthy controls. *Journal of Clinical Psychiatry*, **56**, 560–568.

Hathaway, S. R. & McKinley, J. C. (1940). A multiphasic personality schedule (Minnesota): construction of the schedule. *Journal of Psychology*, **10**, 249–254.

Hyler, S. E., Skodol, A. E., Kellman, H. D., *et al* (1990) Validity of the Personality Disorder Questionnaire – revised: comparison with two structured interviews. *American Journal of Psychiatry*, **147**, 1043–1048.

Langbehn, D. R., Pfohl, B. M., Reynolds, S. *et al* (1999) The Iowa personality disorder screen: development and preliminary validation of a brief screening interview. *Journal of Personality Disorders*, **13**, 75–89.

Livesley, W. J., Jang, K. L. & Vernon, P. A. (1998) Phenotypic and genetic structure of traits delineating personality disorder. *Archives of General Psychiatry*, **55**, 941–48.

Loranger, A.W., Susman, V. L., Oldham, J. M., *et al* (1985) *Personality Disorder Examination (PDE). A Structured Interview for DSM–III–R and ICD–9 Personality Disorders. WHOI ADAMHA Pilot Version*. White Plains, NY: New York Hospital, Comell Medical Center.

Mann, A. H., Jenkins, R., Cutting, J. C., *et al* (1981) The development and use of a standardised assessment of abnormal personality. *Psychological Medicine*, **11**, 839–847.

Millon, T. (1982) *Millon Clinical Multiaxial Inventory* (2nd edn). Minneapolis: Interpretative Scoring System.

Modestin, J. & Puhan, A. (2000) Comparison of assessments of personality disorder by patients and informants. *Psychopathology*, **33**, 265–270.

Moran, P., Leese, M, Lee, T., *et al* (2003) Standardised Assessment of Personality – Abbreviated Scale (SAPAS): preliminary validation of a brief scale for personality disorder. *British Journal of Psychiatry*, **183**, 228–232.

Mulder, R. T. & Joyce, P. R. (1997) Temperament and the structure of personality disorder symptoms. *Psychological Medicine*, **27**, 99–106.

Pfohl, B., Stangi, D. & Zimmerman, M. (1983) *Structured Interview for DSM–III Personality* (SIDP). Iowa City: University of Iowa.

Phillips, K. A., Gunderson, J. G., Triebwasser, J., *et al* (1998) Reliability and validity of depressive personality disorder. *American Journal of Psychiatry*, **155**, 1044–1048.

Sara, G., Raven, P. & Mann, A. (1996) A comparison of DSM–III–R and ICD–10 personality criteria in an out-patient population. *Psychological Medicine*, **26**, 151–160.

Schneider, K. (1923) [Die psychopathischen Personlichkeiten.] Vienna: Deuticke.

Schneider, K. (1950) *Psychopathic Personalities for Modern Classificatory Schemes* (9th edn). London: Cassell.

Spitzer, R. L., Williams, J. & Gibbon, M. (1987) *Structured Clinical Interview for DSM–III–R (SCID–II)*. New York: Biometrics Research, New York State Psychiatric Institute.

Thompson, D. J. & Goldberg, D. (1987) Hysterical personality disorder. The process of diagnosis in clinical and experimental settings. *British Journal of Psychiatry*, **150**, 241–245.

Tyrer, P. (2002) Practice guidelines for the treatment of borderline personality disorder: a bridge too far. *Journal of Personality Disorders*, **16**, 113–118.

Tyrer, P. (2005) Deconstructing personality disorder. *Quarterly Journal of Mental Health*, **1**, 20–24.

Tyrer P, & Alexander J. (1979) Classification of personality disorder. *British Journal of Psychiatry*, **135**, 163–167.

Widiger, T. A. & Simonsen, E. (2005) Alternative dimensional models of personality disorder: finding a common ground. *Journal of Personality Disorders*, **19**, 110–130.

World Health Organization (1992) ICD–10 *Classification of Diseases and Related Health Problems* (ICD–10). Geneva: WHO

Zanarini, M. C., Frankenburg, F. R., Sickel, A. E., *et al* (1994) *Diagnostic Interview for DSM–IV Personality Disorders* (DIPD–IV). Massachusetts: McLean Hospital, 115 Mill Street, Belmont.

Zimmerman, M. (1994) Diagnosing personality disorders: a review of issues and research methods. *Archives of General Psychiatry*, **511**, 225–245.

Appendix I
Psychiatric syndromes

Blocq's disease

Also known as astasia-abasia. This is the inability to walk or stand in a normal manner. The gait is bizarre and is not suggestive of any organic lesion. It is often characterised by swaying and almost falling, with recovery at the last moment. It is a conversion symptom (dissociative motor disorder in ICD–10 and conversion disorder in DSM–IV).

Briquet's syndrome

Now called somatisation disorder, Briquet's syndrome is a condition in which there are multiple physical complaints, in several systems, for which no physical cause is found. It begins usually before the age of 30 years, runs a chronic course and is associated with frequent medical contact. The term was used synonymously with St Louis hysteria, although conversion or dissociative features are rare.

Capgras syndrome

An uncommon syndrome in which the patient believes that a person to whom they are close, usually a family member, has been replaced by an exact double. The underlying psychopathology is delusional misidentification rather than a hallucinatory experience. Other related delusional misidentification syndromes also exist. These include Fregoli syndrome (see below), the syndrome of intermetamorphosis and the syndrome of subjective doubles. The syndrome of intermetamorphosis is characterised by delusions that people have swapped identities while maintaining the same appearance, so it is not just a disguise but a total transformation that is psychological as well as physical. The syndrome of subjective doubles is characterised by the delusional belief that the patient has a double or *doppelganger*.

In reduplicative paramnesia there is a delusional belief that identical places and events exist.

Charles-Bonnet syndrome

This is a syndrome of visual hallucinations without any other psychotic features or any evidence of psychiatric disorder. It is associated with visual impairment. The content of the hallucinations varies from straight lines to complex pictures of people and buildings. They may be enjoyable or distressing. Its importance for psychiatrists lies in not making an erroneous diagnosis of a psychiatric disorder.

Cotard syndrome

A delusion in which the person believes that they are dead. It may be accompanied by delusions that they are rotting, smell malodorous or that parts of the body do not exist (nihilistic delusions). The individual may also be deluded that they have no head, that they have a shadow and cannot see themselves in the mirror. SCAN (World Health Organization, 1998) regards it as a psychotic form of derealisation or depersonalisation and refers to these symptoms as delusions of depresonalisation or derealisation.

Couvade syndrome

This is an abnormality of the experience of self in which a spouse also complains of obstetric symptoms during his partner's pregnancy and parturition. The condition usually arises in the second and third trimester and as well as complaining of symptoms such as nausea, abdominal pain, toothache, food cravings, etc, there is a preoccupation with the spouse's condition. The person is not delusional since he does not believe he is pregnant and it is more akin to a conversion disorder in which his anxieties about his wife's pregnancy are converted into physical symptoms. There is some evidence that it is increasing in frequency owing to the greater role that men have in pregnancy and childbirth in the Western world. It is thus viewed by some not as a conversion disorder per se, but as a manifestation of a deep empathy between the man and his partner. Others believe that it is an attempt to empathise with the foetus or an ambivalence about parenthood. Gross forms of the disorder, in which the man actually experiences the pain of delivery, are rare.

'Culture-bound' disorders

Although known as 'culture-bound' disorders, in recent years, it has become apparent that many of these disorders occur in a variety of cultural settings and may be related to a greater or lesser extent to other diagnostic categories (such as anxiety disorders or psychosis). Koro is an anxiety-related syndrome centred on the idea that the penis is shrinking into the abdomen and that this will be followed by death. Though traditionally only associated with specific cultural settings, such as the Malay culture in Singapore, Koro is now also reported in Western Europe and elsewhere. Other syndromes include Amok (a dissociative or depressive disorder associated with South-East Asia), Dhat syndrome (a psychosexual disorder associated with Asia), Windigo (a depressive condition with the delusion that one has become cannabilistic, seen in Native Americans) and Susto (an anxiety disorder related to the loss of soul, seen in South and Central America). Latah, consisting of startle-induced disorganisation, automatic obedience, echopraxia and hypersuggestability, occurs in South-East Asia while Piblokto, found among Eskimos, presents with attacks of screaming, crying and running naked through the snow.

De Clerambault's syndrome or erotomania	This is a condition in which the patient, often a single woman, believes than an exalted person is in love with her. Usually the supposed lover is inaccessible, for example a famous television performer whom she only sees while watching the television. The patient may believe that the object of her love is presently unable to make his feelings known to her, for various reasons, and she may feel that the subject cannot live happily without her. Sometimes the patient may stalk or pester the object of her desires. Sometimes this is regarded as a paradoxical proof of love. Erotomania may also be a feature of paranoid schizophrenia.
Diogenes syndrome	This is characterised by gross self-neglect, especially among elderly reclusive persons, though not always. They are often wealthy and intelligent and about 50% have no psychiatric illness, although they have a history of being reclusive and may have paranoid personality disorder. Some authorities believe that this is an end-stage personality disorder. The remainder have schizophrenia or dementia. As well as neglect the person may live in squalour, refuse any offers of help and sometimes hoard rubbish

(syllogomania) yet be seemingly unconcerned about their situation.

Ekbom's syndrome — Also known as restless legs syndrome, this is a common sensorimotor disorder with a prevalence of 1–5%. Patients complain of unpleasant sensations experienced predominantly in the legs and rarely in the arms. The symptoms occur only at rest and become more pronounced in the evening or at night. There is often a strong urge to move the limbs, resulting in only temporary relief of symptoms. It is characterised by periodic leg movements during sleep and these may interfere with sleep onset. Equally common in men and women, its prevalence increases with increasing age. In some it may be familial.

Fregoli syndrome — One of the delusional misidentification syndromes in which it is believed that various people whom the subject meets are really the same person, in disguise. For example, a patient believed that her neighbour could change his appearance, clothes and even his sex at will so as to spy on her.

Ganser syndrome — This syndrome was first described in 1898 when it occurred in four criminals. It continues to have an association with prisoners and army personnel under severe stress, such as when awaiting trial or going to war. The person seems to mimic their own view of what constitutes severe psychiatric illness and so it is characterised by approximate answers (an answer indicating that the question is understood but the answer is incorrect and absurd) or *vorbeireden*, clouding of consciousness with disorientation, hallucinations (either auditory or visual) and amnesia for the period during the episode. Perseveration, exholalia, echopraxia and hysterical paralysis may also be observed and symptoms are worse when the patient is being observed. It is associated with a recent history of head injury or severe emotional stress and resolves very quickly but may be followed by major depression. Personality disorder is a risk factor. It has variously been formulated as a factitious disorder, as a form of malingering, a hysterical condition (hence the name hysterical pseudodementia), one that has an organic basis or a reactive psychosis (Ungvari & Mullen, 1997).

Korsakoff's syndrome	This is an amnestic disorder caused by thiamine deficiency that occurs in chronic alcohol misuse. It is characterised by impairment of recent memory, apathy and confabulation to fill in the gaps in memory.
Othello syndrome	Also called morbid jealousy, this is a delusional belief or overvalued idea that one's spouse/partner is being unfaithful. Occurring in men more than women, it may be present on its own or as a symptom of schizophrenia, alcohol abuse or cocaine abuse. It is highly dangerous and may lead to stalking, searching or sometimes violence.
Munchausen's syndrome	Also known as hospital addiction, this belongs to the category of factitious disorders. It is characterised by repeated presentations for hospital treatment of an apparent acute illness with plausible symptoms and a dramatic history, all of which are false. The person may also self-injure so as to gain admission to hospital. The disorder first appeared in the psychiatric literature in the 1950s. Unlike malingering, there does not appear to be any secondary gain such as money. Rather the motivation seems to be to assume the role of patient and be cared for.
Munchausen's syndrome by proxy	First named in 1976, this is a controversial diagnosis, in which a person, usually a mother but not exclusively so, intentionally induces or fabricates an illness in a child or other person under their care. Thus they use the child (or other person) to fulfil their need to step into the sick role. Also called Polle syndrome, after the only child of Baron Von Munchausen who died aged 1 year, its controversy stems from the presumption about the underpinning motivation, from the features said to be diagnostic of the disorder and from inadequate validation. Convictions based on this diagnosis have also recently been overturned in the courts in Britain.

References

Ungvari, G. S. & Mullen, P. E. (1997) Reactive Psychosis. In *Troublesome disguises: Underdiagnosed Psychiatric Syndromes* (eds D. Bhugra & A. Munro), pp. 52–90. Oxford: Blackwell Science.

World Health Organization (1998) *Schedules for Clinical Assessment in Neuropsychiatry.* Geneva: WHO.

Appendix II
Defences and distortions

Defence mechanisms

These are the techniques used by the psyche to protect itself from overwhelming anxiety or stress. These are not entities in themselves, but explanations derived originally from psychoanalysis to explain symptoms and behaviour. The list below is not exhaustive but describes those most commonly seen in practice.

Altruism	Describes the mechanism of satisfying one's own needs through the lives of others. For example, the man who wished he had become a doctor may 'push' his family into this career and blame himself if they do not fulfil his expectations.
Denial	Defined as the expressed refusal to acknowledge a threatening reality (for example, 'it can't happen here'). It is of relevance especially to those with serious physical illnesses, where the patient denies being told of the presence of any illness in themselves or their loved ones. It may persist despite constant reiteration of the facts. The term denial is often used, inappropriately, for the knowing or conscious avoidance of painful topics or thoughts.
Displacement	The process by which interest and/or emotion is shifted from one object onto another less-threatening one, so that the latter replaces the former. Thus the person who loses a child in a road accident and thereafter devotes themselves tirelessly to campaigning against dangerous driving is exhibiting this defence. From a psychological perspective, the affect that attached to the child is replaced by the affect attached to the ideals of the campaign. More prosaically, the person who is having problems at work may displace the

	anger felt for their boss onto their family by displaying irritability and moodiness at home, or a spinster may accumulate numerous cats rather than children.
Idealisation	The ascribing of omnipotence to another person or organisation (for example, 'you will save me').
Identification with the aggressor	Observed where the victim begins to assume the qualities or faults of the opponent. This may show itself as the battered wife believing she deserves to be beaten and justifying her husband's aggression to her. The 'Stockholm syndrome' is another example (Favaro *et al*, 2000).
Projection	The defence against unpalatable anxieties, impulses or attributes in one's own psyche, which are attributed to an external origin. For example, the person who attributes indecision to others may be unconsciously projecting their own indecisiveness. Thus internal threats become externalised and then are easier to handle.
Projective identification	A defence in which first an aspect of self is projected onto someone else. The projector tries to coerce the recipient to identify with what has been projected and both feel a sense of union. This may result in the recipient behaving in a manner similar to the projector.
Rationalisation	Involves finding excuses that will justify unacceptable behaviours when self-esteem is threatened, for example 'it was OK for me to behave as I did because he hit me first'.
Reaction formation	Refers to the denial of an unacceptable impulse and the adoption of the opposing behaviour. This can lead to morality crusades or a prurient interest in the subject.
Repression	Characterised by the unconscious forgetting of painful ideas or impulses in order to protect the psyche; it overlaps with denial.
Somatosensory amplification	The tendency to experience bodily sensations as unusually intense or distressing (Barsky, 1992) and this is thought to underpin somatisation and the somatoform disorders.
Splitting	Found most frequently in those with borderline personality disorder, occurs when people, both past and present, are divided into their polar opposites. Thus they are regarded either as perfect or deeply flawed, exclusively nurturing or rejecting.

Sublimation | The transfer of unacceptable impulses or urges onto more acceptable alternatives, for example anger being transferred onto political activism. There were suggestions that Freud sublimated his sexual urges by the pursuit of science. Sublimation is similar to displacement.

Cognitive distortions

Cognitive distortions are errors in thinking that impinge upon the person's view of themselves, of other people and of their own future. The following have been adapted from Burns (1990) and from Ellis & Grieger (1986).

All-or-nothing thinking | Things are seen in black and white; if performance falls short of perfect, the person regards themself as a total failure, for example if a person fails to be promoted to the post they desperately wanted, they believe they will never be promoted and that their career is in ruins.

Approval-seeking | You must be approved of and loved all the time and if not then life is terrible. This results in compromising your needs so as to gain the approval others.

Comparison | You constantly compare yourself to others with little information or on the basis of an isolated event; so you feel either superior or inferior.

Disqualifying positive | You reject positive experiences by insisting they 'don't count' for some reason or other. In this way you can maintain a negative belief that is contradicted by your everyday experiences; for example, a pleasant employee pays you a compliment and you say it is in order to get a good reference. This takes the joy out of living and leaves you feeling unrewarded.

Emotional reasoning | You assume that your negative emotions necessarily reflect the way things really are: 'I feel it, therefore it must be true'. For example, you look at the large volume of work and feel overwhelmed; you conclude there is no point in even trying.

Fallacy of fairness | You judge a negative event as unfair when it isn't an issue of justice; for example, you live a healthy lifestyle yet you become ill and think 'how unfair'. Of course people get ill regardless of their lifestyle.

Jumping to conclusions | You make a negative interpretation even though there are no definite facts that convincingly support your conclusion. Two types are found:
• Mind reading: you automatically draw a negative conclusion without facts to support it; for example,

your daughter won't tidy her room and you believe it is because she is deliberately trying to wind you up.

- The fortune-teller error: you can predict that things will turn out badly, and you feel convinced that your prediction is a fait accompli; for example, you decide not to ask someone for a date because you know they'll refuse anyway.

Labelling mislabelling	This is an extreme form of overgeneralisation; and instead of describing your error, you attach a negative label to yourself; for example, you break your diet and say 'I'm a weak-willed slob'. When somebody else's behaviour annoys you, you attach a negative label to them – 'they're a selfish pig'. Mislabelling involves describing an event with language that is highly coloured and emotionally loaded.
Magnification (catastrophising) minimisation	You focus on the worst possible outcome and overestimate the probability that it will happen (magnification) or you inappropriately shrink the importance of an attribute or event (minimisation). This is also called the 'binocular trick'. For example, you have a pain in your head and you think it is cancer (magnification) or you are playing tennis and lose the first set but your game picks up and you win. When others compliment you, you say it was just chance that you won as you played badly (minimisation). Or 'it doesn't matter that my TV licence is due. It can wait for another while' (minimisation).
Mental filtering/ selective perception	You pick out a single negative detail and dwell on it exclusively, while ignoring all the rest, so that your vision of all reality becomes darkened. For example, a driver waves you into a traffic lane, but later when another car cuts-in in front of you, you believe that all drivers are rude and thoughtless. Alternatively, for women, you are at a party and everybody tells you that you look glamorous but then somebody suggests that you should put colour in your hair and you feel distraught and your evening is ruined.
Overgeneralisation	One takes a single negative event and makes a general rule out of it without ever testing this rule. Words such as 'always', 'never', 'everybody' permeate the thinking – 'I'm always messing things up; 'I never get anything right; Everybody is sick of me'; or the shy person who, when ignored by one person, sees no point in trying to meet other people because 'everybody is out for themselves'.

Perfectionism	You and others must be perfect and when this does not happen you become upset even if the matter is unimportant.
Personalisation	You see yourself as the cause of some negative external event, which in fact you were not primarily responsible for, for example blaming yourself when your child is misbehaving at school. The emotional consequence is guilt.
Reductionism	You fail to see the complex causes or the potential benefits of a situation. Instead you reduce it to a simple cause and a simple consequence. Your son has not got the points for university and you think he will never be a success in life or that the experience may lead to him working harder for the next exam.
Self-rightous cognitions	People should always do what you think is right and if they don't they are wrong and should be punished. These people are critical of others and see them as 'stupid', 'bad', etc.
Should statements	You try to motivate yourself with should and shouldn't, must and ought, as if you had to be punished before you could be expected to do anything; the emotional consequences are guilt. When you direct should statements towards others, you feel anger, frustration, and resentment. For example, you are kept waiting in your psychiatrist's waiting room and you think to yourself, 'he should be more considerate. I've had to rush to get here'. In fact, he's dealing with an emergency. This has also been termed 'musterbation' by Albert Ellis, the psychotherapist who developed rational emotive behaviour therapy.
'Woe is me'	You see yourself as a victim even when the situation is ordinary. For example, you have to go to the shop because you have run out of milk. You see this as a huge challenge and fail to take responsibility because you couldn't be bothered getting it when you were shopping earlier in the day.

Acknowledgement

The authors thank Mr Odhran McCarthy, Senior Clinical Psychologist, Mater Misericordiae Hospital, Dublin, Ireland, for his assistance in proof reading this appendix.

References

Barsky, A. J. (1992) Amplification, somatization and the somatoform disorders. *Psychosomatics*, **33**, 28–34.

Burns, D. (1990) *Feeling Good. The New Mood Therapy*. New York: New American Library.

Ellis, A. & Grieger, R. (1986) *Handbook of Rational–Emotive Therapy*. 2. New York: Springer.

Favaro, A., Degortes, D., Colombo, G., *et al* (2000) The effects of trauma among kidnap victims in Sardinia, Italy. *Psychological Medicine*, **30**, 975–980.

Index

Compiled by Linda English